INSTANT
Teaching Tools

for the
New Millennium

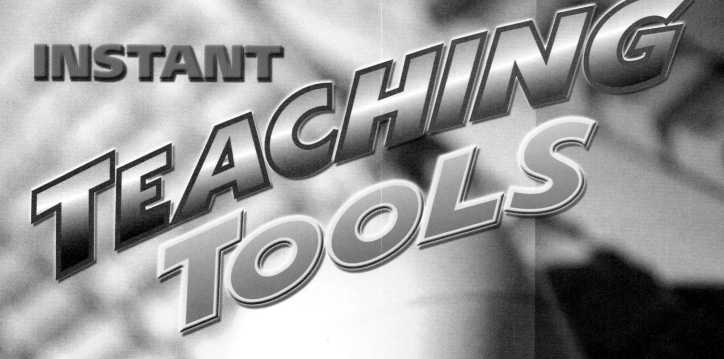

INSTANT TEACHING TOOLS

for the New Millennium

Michele L. Deck, MEd, RN, BSN, LCCE, FACCE

President and Chief Executive Officer, G.A.M.E.S.
Chief Executive Officer, Tool Thyme for Trainers
Metairie, Louisiana

Mosby

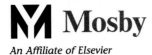

An Affiliate of Elsevier

11830 Westline Industrial Drive
St. Louis, Missouri 63146

INSTANT TEACHING TOOLS FOR THE NEW MILLENNIUM

ISBN: 0-323-02666-4

First Edition 2004.

Senior Editor: Yvonne Alexopoulos
Associate Developmental Editor: Kristin Hebberd
Publishing Services Manager: Catherine Jackson

Printed in the United States of America

Last digit is print number: 9 8 7 6 5 4 3 2 1

CONTRIBUTORS

Gina M. Ankner, MSN, RN, CS-ANP
Faculty Member
University of Massachusetts Dartmouth
College of Nursing
Dartmouth, MA

Jeri Ashley, RN, MSN, AOCN, CCRC
Supportive Oncology Services, Inc.
Memphis, TN

Sherry Blanchard, RN
Educator
Great River Medical Center
West Burlington, IA

Susan Bosold, MS, MA, RN
Assistant Professor of Nursing
Grand Valley State University
Grand Rapids, MI

Cheryl Burdette, MEd, RN
Centra Health
Lynchburg, VA

Gino Chisari, RN, MSN
Malden, MA

Erin Davis, MS, MEd, RRT
Director of Clinical Education
Program in Respiratory Care
Ochsner School of Allied Health Sciences
New Orleans, LA

Cecelia Deslauriers, RN, CLC,
 IBCLC, BS
Libertyville, IL

Martin Isganitis, BS
Decatur, GA

Vivian Jefferson, RN, MSN
Director of Education
Morehead Memorial Hospital
Eden, NC

Jennifer Kadis, MSN, RN, CPAN
Clinical Nurse Specialist, Surgical Services
Memorial Hospital West
Pembrokes Pines, FL

Mary LaBiche, MEd, RRT
Program Director
Program in Respiratory Care
Ochsner School of Allied Health Sciences
New Orleans, LA

Donna McHenry, NREMT-P
Director of EMS Education and
 Development
Porter Memorial
Valparaiso, IN

Margaret O'Hara, RN, MSN
Assistant Coordinator
Youville Hospital & Rehabilitation Center
School of Practical Nursing
Cambridge, MA

Bernadette Price, RN, MSN
Associate Professor
Purdue University, Calumet
Schereville, IN

Chris Reid, RN, MSN
Associate Professor
Purdue University, Calumet
Schereville, IN

Rhonda Scott-Foertsh, RN, BSN
Practical Nursing Instructor
Juniata-Mifflin Counties Area
 Vocational-Technical School
Practical Nursing Department
Lewistown, PA

JoAnn Segarra, RN, BSN, CNOR
Nurse Clinician
Memorial Hospital West
Pembrokes Pines, FL

Sandra Stokes, RN
Human Resource Development Consultant
UNC Health Care
Chapel Hill, NC

Laura Sumner, MEd, MBA, RN, ONC
Clinical Educator
Department of Nursing
Massachusetts General Hospital
The Center for Clinical & Professional
 Development
Boston, MA

Iris Trahan, RN, BSN, CCRN
Training Specialist
Ochsner Clinic Foundation
East Jefferson General Hospital
New Orleans, LA

Sandy Wilbanks, RN, BSN, CDE
Kawkawlin, MI

PREFACE

The transition from professional to educator is an exciting one! It is filled with wonder and the awesome power of influencing the future. It is filled with lots of hard work and much joy. Education ranges from teaching some-one life-saving skills to recognizing the power of personal connections and building relationships. Many times it is assumed that teaching involves telling the learners everything you know about a topic, simply being a source of information. Many professionals have this gift of knowledge before they begin teaching others, and they think that knowledge is all that is nec-essary. They are very surprised when they first try to teach something the learners already know. They suddenly find that teaching requires an entirely different set of skills altogether! It requires knowing ways to teach that are involving and interactive, ways that gain and keep the learners' attention. It requires planning for reflection time and provides time for learners to prac-tice skills. Teaching involves getting the learners to believe that they can remember the information and achieve success through the skills they have learned from you. To achieve these results, it takes a desire to be a learner yourself and the courage to try new and different approaches to teaching. Some educators learn their teaching skills through trial and error. This process can be a long and difficult one and filled with frustration. For those of us who are lucky, we find someone to mentor us and to show us the way. We don't have to "reinvent the wheel."

The purpose of *Instant Teaching Tools for the New Millennium* is to be a men-toring resource for those educators who use it. It offers many new ideas on how to approach a topic, as well as ideas that are mandated and repeated annually. Seasoned educators have already tried these approaches and know that they produce successful outcomes. They have generously shared them here so that you may benefit from their experiences. Take advantage of the offer and try a few. You will be surprised at the results. Learning time will be less, and the learner's ability to remember will be higher. People will enjoy the process of learning, and you will too. Even serious topics can be taught in joyful ways.

For those of you who have seen and done it all in education, I offer this book as a way to rejuvenate your energy and creativity. Each of us needs to recharge our batteries with some new methods and materials each year to keep ourselves interested and enthusiastic about teaching. If we become bored with the process of teaching, we lose the reason to do it. After all, it may be the first time a learner ever hears it, even when it is the 500th time you have taught it. A new learner deserves to experience the same positive outcome that the first learner received from you. These new approaches can re-energize repetitive classes.

The ideas are to be used and adapted as you see fit. With the CD-ROM, activity pages can be printed or placed on intranets or in Internet courses, and ideas can be immediately implemented in a class.

In a world of high-tech instant access to information, there is a very real need for human connection. Make your teaching experiences a part of reaching out and touching others, and you will find a terrific bonus in your job. You will find a satisfaction in and a desire to really help others. You will become a part of the wondrous circle of learning and the circle of life. You will be valued for your wisdom and your experience. I hope *Instant Teaching Tools for the New Millennium* will be a part of the road map in your journey! I have found many blessings in the teaching of others. I hope you will feel a part of that spirit too. Good luck, and welcome to the circle. I hope our paths cross soon!

—Michele Deck

ACKNOWLEDGMENTS

I have been so blessed by the spirit of so many wonderful people who have come into my life. I'd first like to thank everyone at Elsevier who has made this third book a reality. Thanks to Yvonne Alexopoulos, my terrific editor, who trusted my unusual vision for this book and has been both adventurous and determined every step of the way. Thanks also to Kristin Hebberd, my developmental editor, who has been patient in tracking me down and waiting for me to call or email from the farthest reaches of my travels. Thanks finally to Julie Nebel, who handled all the paperwork and kept up with me about all the details. Their vision has made this book a smooth and fun adventure.

I'd like to thank the many talented and generous health care educators and nursing faculty I have met over the last 14 years of full-time travel. It is so nice to meet creative people who have pioneered new ways of teaching when others around them may all be shaking their heads. I am inspired by these educators' efforts to always find a better way to teach critical content. It is noble to create and mentor the generation of health care providers who will be taking care of us in the future. I personally want them to be the "cream of the crop." I'm sure you do as well. Teaching others to be top thinkers, problem solvers, doers, and mentors is the whole point of educating others.

Thank you to the professional colleagues who have contributed their terrific works to this book. Thanks to Vivian, Susan, Sherry, Sandra, Chris, Bernadette, Gina, Rhonda, Sandy, Margaret, Gino, Laura, Iris, Martin, Cheryl, Cecelia, Donna, Jeri, Jennifer, JoAnn, Erin, and Mary. Thank you for your generosity in sharing these ideas with everyone who reads this book. Your efforts are amazing and are to be applauded!

Thanks also to my family for your support and love. Two of my sisters have volunteered countless hours at conferences, presentations, and exhibits. My sister Cindy Baune is the best international sales director I know, able to communicate with a variety of people who don't speak English. She has given me countless hours of business and life advice. My sister Mary Ann Lafayette delights me with her talent for adding a group of numbers in her head while remembering every number I have forgotten. She is also a talented director of communications; she can gather a crowd at breakfast and know everyone's name in the time it takes to buy a muffin! Both Cindy and Mary Ann have left their own businesses at the drop of a hat to help me out with mine. Thanks also to my other two sisters—Kathy Bosworth, who taught me about miracles through prayer, and Pat Schonacher, who gave me the gift of my master's degree. Thank you for being the best people in the world, who just happen to be my sisters.

There are so many people who have mentored me over the years. Thanks to Jeanne Silva, Heather Banton, Lori Backer, Doug McCallum, Lynn Solem, and Pat and Bob Bender. You listened to my panicked phone calls at all hours of the day and night, applied Velcro to props with me, found odd pasta for auctions, stayed up looking for a hidden, ringing alarm, cried behind flipcharts, laughed at goofy things with me, and prayed for and counseled me in the belief in the abundance of God. Thank you for always answering my questions and supporting all my efforts. I am truly blessed by your love and support.

All of *Instant Teaching Tools for the New Millennium* and my travels would not be possible without the support of my wonderful husband and partner, Brian. Thank you for listening from far-off cities, telling me to "buck up" when necessary, and for making me laugh so often. The first 25 years have flown by! The best blessings I have ever received are my three beautiful daughters, Melanie, Melissa, and Brittany. I am so proud that you are strong, independent, smart women with a host of talents that shine. Thank you for your unconditional love and continuing inspiration and for recognizing that I can be a "big cheese ball." May your careers and personal lives continue to be a source of unending joy to you as you have been to me.

—*Michele Deck*

ABOUT THE AUTHOR

Michele L. Deck, MEd, RN, BSN, LCCE, FACCE

Michele Deck, an internationally renowned presenter, author, and educator, is the co-founder, president, and chief executive officer of G.A.M.E.S., a company that offers seminars to organizations that specialize in adult learning and interactive teaching methods. She is also the founder and CEO of Tool Thyme for Trainers, a company that provides the most innovative and creative presentation tools available worldwide to educators. Thousands of people from Australia to Scotland and from Canada to Taiwan have gained valuable expertise in adult education and training from her presentations. Some of her books include *Instant Teaching Tools for Health Care Educators; More Instant Teaching Tools for Health Care Educators; Presenter's Survival Kit; It's a Jungle Out There!; Getting Adults Motivated, Enthusiastic, and Satisfied; Getting Adults Motivated, Enthusiastic, and Satisfied,* volume two; *The Presenter's E-Z Graphics Kit: for the Artistically Challenged; Live to Train Another Day; and The First Aid Idea Kit,* parts 1 and 2.

Michele is known for her innovative teaching methods in the field of health care education and training. She has been training educators and trainers full time for the last 17 years. She has acted as a consultant to Creative Training Techniques International, Inc., from 1988 to 1999, and was named Best Overall Trainer by the Creative Training Techniques Companies. She has won the prestigious Excellence in Nursing award, has been selected as one of the Great 100 Nurses in Louisiana, and was also elected to the Sigma Theta Tau National Nursing Honor Society. The National Nursing Staff Development Organization named her the recipient of the prestigious Belinda Puetz award in 2000.

Michele consistently receives high evaluations as a result of her fun, informative, and idea-filled sessions. She has facilitated more than 500 learning sessions on a variety of topics. Michele has made presentations at many national and international conferences. Clients include Dun and Bradstreet, Hibernia National Bank, Bayley and Bender, Bank One, Barnett Bank, United Parcel Service, Häagen Dazs Ice Cream, Informix, U.S. Coast Guard Academy, Abbott Labs, Eli Lilly, Boston Pizza, Southern Nuclear, and Oxford Shirt Company. Michele's health care clients have included the American Association of Critical Care Nurses, the National Association of Operating Room Nurses, the National Association of Orthopedic Nurses, the American Association of Office Nurses, the Emergency Nurses Association, the American Association of Occupational Health Nurses, the American Association of Diabetes Educators, Sanofi Pharmaceuticals, Lovelace Health Services, the Vermont Cardiac Network, the American Red Cross, SCA Hygiene Products–Eli Lilly, the Louisiana Department of Health and Hospitals, and the Naval School of Health Sciences.

CONTENTS

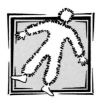
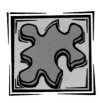
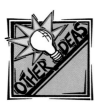

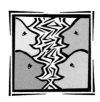
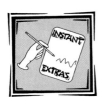

PART 1
Challenges We Share

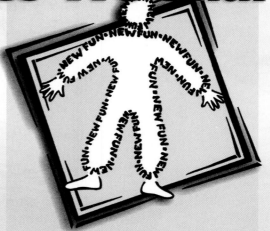

Challenges We Share

Multiple Roles for Those Who Educate

Today, educators are faced with many interesting and baffling challenges. They are expected to meet the learning needs of a wide variety of people on just about any topic and sometimes to become a model or performance coach and master problem solver. Some educators are faced with all these responsibilities while doing another full-time job in which education and training is just a small part. I admire and respect the health care educators who teach fellow staff, allied health professionals, and nursing students, because they must instruct students in the complexities of critical thinking. They also work with learners of different ages, with different histories, cultures, and job descriptions, as well as different stressors and priorities. "Teachnology" is also a factor in their work. Many educators are teaching in both the virtual and real world. It is for these educators that I have collected such an eclectic mix of teaching ideas to share in this book.

Many Generations in the Classroom and Job Market

Four different generations are in the job market and in health care education programs today. The first group is the *Traditionalists,* born before 1946. This group of people has seen history being made every day and has their own perspective on education and on-the-job learning. They prefer to receive their information verbally with a face-to-face encounter. As a group they do not want to be involved with "teachnology" any more than is necessary. Traditionalists are very singular in focus and do not like to multitask. They also hate to be part of any waste of resources. They respect and follow those who have titles of authority without questioning style or ability, they like to take their time, and they have learned to stop and appreciate all life has brought them.

Working with the Traditionalists are the *Baby Boomers,* born from 1946 until 1960. This is the highly overworked generation, with the belief that their jobs define their identities. This is also the first generation that thought they could "have it all," acting as super parents and super community members while working much more than 40 hours a week. They never hesitated to stay late and arrive early at work. This group also shared a love-hate relationship with those in authority, and its members have learned to wait out hard times, often saying, "Just wait—things will get better when that person leaves in a year." They talk about "circles" and wait for proof of them. This group has maintained a hectic pace for a number of years and has trouble slowing down. They can use "teachnology" but if offered a choice would prefer to learn something relevant in a live classroom where they can "see" it. Baby Boomers like to both hear and see information. This group represents more than 75% of the middle and upper management in health care today. Younger workers who do not share their singular focus on job and career sometimes confuse and confound their Baby Boomer managers.

Members of *Generation X* (Gen Xers), born between 1961 and 1980, are also in the workplace. This is the generation that was raised to be independent; many were latchkey kids who were left alone after school while their parents were at work. This group is also reluctant to commit in both their personal and professional lives. They have watched their parents' relationships fall apart (possibly because of lack of balance) and seen businesses with long histories fail. They know how to relax, and many see work as just a means to an end—not the cornerstone of their identity. This group has a talent for dealing with change at a rapid pace and for being "techno savvy." They will work to better their skills; when the work conditions get bad, they do not hesitate to leave and go somewhere else. They follow people who are competent and excellent at their jobs, even if those people do not hold a title. They do not like people to waste their time with teaching information that is "nice to know." They want to learn about things relevant to them, and they like to learn rapidly and conveniently in the most visual way possible. This is one of the groups driving the internet/intranet learning format. They have grown up with the media all around them and expect to be entertained while learning.

Many of us are starting to see the arrival of the *Generation Y* (Gen Yers). This is the generation born between 1981 and 2002. They are seeking a more traditional life and commitment to family than the Gen Xers. Many of them are marrying early and having families young. This group is completely "techno ready." (If you have a technological glitch, find a 12 year old to solve it!) This group is also amazing in its short attention span and desire to learn in sound bites in a technological or hands-on format. This group is the most ethnically diverse the United States has ever known and is sure to make its mark on the world. Their numbers are large, and they seem to have money to spend; therefore marketing and the media are beginning to target this group by appealing to them in new and different ways. This is also the Internet age learner who can access any source of information in minutes and expects learning to follow that pattern. They are not listeners—but seers and doers. They love kinesthetic learning experiences and lose interest very quickly when bored.

Television and the Media's Influence

I like to refer to the mass of these four different generations as the *television generation learners*. Many people in all four of these groups have been unconsciously conditioned by television to expect their learning to be highly visual, entertaining, and broken up into manageable sound bites. I often ask educators if they recognize these learners in their classes. You can tell who they are by seeing signs and symptoms that they are on a "pinball trip" in class. Their bodies may be in the seat, but their brains are focusing on a number of different topics unrelated to the class topic. They are mentally pinging from place to place in their minds, just as a pinball travels through a game machine, hitting various obstacles and scoring points.

Getting and Keeping Learner Attention

The following are the five and one half symptoms educators see when their learners are on a pinball trip:

1. *Napjerk:* This is the phenomenon one sees when learners are so relaxed in class they are drifting off to sleep and jump as they move into a deeper state of relaxation.
2. *Pezhead:* Just like a Pez candy dispenser, the learners' heads go back as they lose interest and drift off to sleep.
3. *Bombie:* This learner is the one giving you the blank stare. Their bodies are in the class, but their brains are not. They look like zombies, but by definition zombies do not have a brain. Our learner has a brain, so brain + zombie = bombie.
4. *Prayerful thought:* This is when the learner props his or her chin in their hand while folding the arms to support the weight of the head. The eyes are either closed or looking down. Many people see this stance at religious functions, usually during sermons.
5a. *"Where did that come from?" question:* This happens when you are giving a fabulous explanation of a topic and someone raises his or her hand. You are shocked when he or she asks you a question that has absolutely nothing to do with the topic you were teaching.
5b. *"I just said that" question:* No sooner have the words come from your mouth than this person asks you to repeat what you just said as if he or she has never heard it before.

If you have seen any of the symptoms listed previously, you can be assured that those persons on pinball trips will not be able to remember what you were trying to teach them at that moment. It is a great frustration to realize this, but it is a fact that educators must deal with every day. Physiologic reasons exist for pinball trips. If we understand why they happen, we can prevent them from occurring.

Fast Thinkers

The average speed of speech that an educator can produce is between 110 to 140 words per minute. The average speed of thought of the learner is between 400 to 1000 words per minute. It is as if the educator is walking on a sidewalk, and next to him or her is the learner on a ten-speed bike, wanting to go very fast. Is it possible for someone on a ten-speed to slow down enough to keep up with someone walking on a sidewalk? Yes, it is possible. Is it comfortable? No. Do learners want to slow down for long periods of time? No, again. Therefore the gap gets in the way.

Most learners are able to overcome the gap for about the same amount of time as a television show allows us. The average length of a network television show segment is between 3 and 14 minutes. When you average it out, the length of a show segment is 5 to 6 minutes. Therefore some of our learners have about a 5- to 6-minute attention span.

Refocusing at Intervals

My approach takes this into consideration. Every 5 to 14 minutes, one must refocus the learners and bring them mentally back to the topic. Many people refer to this as "engaging" the learner. It is a process that cycles through good teaching and is absent in boring classes. Refocus the learners when you see pinball trips happening; don't just continue on!

Doing any activity can "reset" the learner's pinball machine and reengage them. I suggest you select activities from this book that make a point about your content and refocus people at the same time. Let's think of it as a two-for-one learning benefit. Using activities does not take more class time, but it does take some preparation time before you arrive. In your preparation, you might copy forms or download ideas from the CD-ROM that accompanies this book. More powerful and memorable teaching can and will occur this way. People cannot drift off to sleep if they are actively involved in the process of learning. That is the ultimate secret of great learning—involving people in a variety of ways often enough to keep their attention.

High Numbers of Visual Learners

To make your content memorable, make it visual. More than 80% of the average population thinks in pictures. When they hear words spoken, their minds play images they can see in their mind's eye. Using visuals, telling stories that create pictures in the learner's mind, and using unusual props can imprint knowledge in visual thinkers.

Varying the Methods

If instructing more than one or two people, use all three categories of teaching methods. For the 10% of the population that is auditory, you will want to tell them the information verbally (or have them repeat what they have learned aloud). In addition, for the majority of learners, you will also want to use a visual approach. You will also want to keep in mind that the kinesthetic, or hands-on doers, must be actively involved in the learning process to stay focused. Statistics show that hands-on doers make up only 10% of the average population, but I find it to be higher in health care (people who are talented with their hands are drawn to a hands-on profession). Therefore I believe that these individuals comprise about 30% of the health care audience. We must ask them to do an activity, take notes, hold an item, or actually do something for them to learn it. As the Gen Yers become more of the learning population, using all three of these educational approaches will be essential.

How to Begin and End Matter

Always remember the importance of primacy and recency in your classes and course design. *Primacy* is the ability to remember the beginning of a list or a presentation, and it is our learner's most memorable experience with us. Therefore their best memory of our class is the first 5 to 14 minutes of the class once we have gained their attention. Some instructors use openers to gain attention, so the best memory begins immediately after the opening is complete. What should you put in this period? The most critical information or the "need to know" should go here. *Recency* is the ability to remember the end of a presentation or list, and it is our learners' second best memory of their time with us. Before I knew about recency, I would lecture until the second my class time was over, or in a module I would print, "The End." Now I prefer to reserve just a few minutes at the end of class to challenge my learners to break up into teams and compete to make the longest list of everything they have learned. In modules, I present my own stealth review of the information at the end. This way learners leave with their second best memory of class being a list of thirty things they learned.

The following figure illustrates how I design content for maximum retention of television generation learners. First, I select how I will gain their attention, interest, and buy in with an opening, represented by the *Open* in the diagram. Then I like to select the way I will close or stealth review content, or skills, represented by the *Close* in the diagram. I like to see the whole process of teaching as a circle, in that information cycles back to where we began once we get to the end.

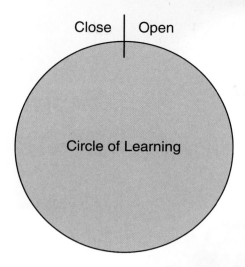

Close | Open

Circle of Learning

Now let's make it interesting! If you were given a deluxe hamburger from a national chain, could you eat it all in one mouthful? Of course not, you would bite it or cut in into manageable pieces. Your content can also be a large volume of information, so you must next decide how to break it into manageable bites. In the following diagram, imagine the content chunks (CC) are the loops falling inside the circle of learning.

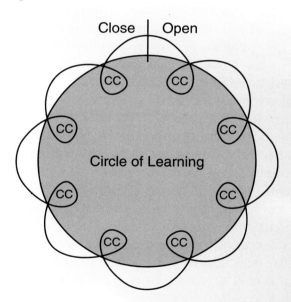

Close | Open

Circle of Learning

Where the loops spill outside of the circle of learning, this is where we refocus people to regain their attention—just as television keeps us interested by interjecting commercials. Learners can be refocused in a variety of ways, including some I'm sure you're using now. Some of those might include a change from lecturing to using media, changing media formats, telling a story, showing a funny cartoon, asking a question, or teaching in another part of the room. The list is endless. This book offers you ideas you can use to open, close, refocus, and increase involvement. The following diagram shows the entire model, with the *R* representing times to "Refocus."

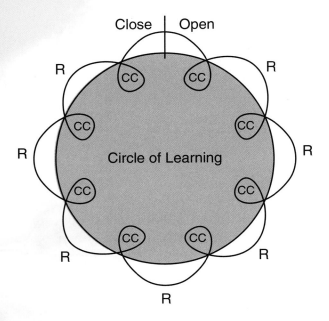

Some educators will say they have no time to restructure all of the classes they have already planned to fit his model. I suggest a practical approach. If you compile a list on an index card of all the possible ways to refocus your learners, you will have a way to quickly adapt classes that need improvement. Conduct the class from your regular outline, and when you look up and see symptoms of a pinball trip occurring, simply insert a refocuser off of your index card. This will allow you to reengage or refocus the learners. Go back to your outline and continue until it is time to insert another refocuser. This way you can take your index card list into any class and use it without restructuring all of your classes. When it is time to plan a new class, you might want to then use the model to plan. This approach can ensure that alert participants who are involved at intervals are receiving information. It also allows you to reach a variety of learners of different backgrounds, ages, cultures, job descriptions, and experience levels. This book presents a variety of ways to teach that diverse mix of learners that educators face everyday with a mountain of information and very little time to teach it.

Icons and Book Format

Each idea in the book has icons to represent important information and easy use. A guide to each of the headings and icons in the book is offered on the following page.

- The **topic** of the activity allows you to find the activity to accomplish your educational goal when looking through the book.

- The *title* of the activity is listed.

- The *name of the person* or *persons* who created the idea, used it first, and generously offered it for your use is listed under the title of the idea.

- The **clock** represents the teaching time needed to conduct the activity.

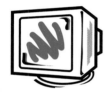

- The **tool box** represents which supplies should be gathered ahead of time.

- In addition, a *preparation* section tells you how to set up the needed items listed in the toolbox.

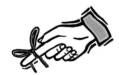

- The *implementation* section tells you in a step-by-step recipe how to conduct the activity.

- The **computer** represents how the Internet/Intranet can be used or adapted to virtual courses.

- The **educator secrets** symbol offers a few more tips learned through the experience of implementing this idea.

The ready-to-use sheets are included with the activities for which they are required. They are also contained within the CD-ROM and can be imported into your teaching documents or audiovideos (AVs) for immediate use; they can also be printed for handouts. In addition, you can create custom, ready-to-use sheets for activities so that you can adapt them to best meet the needs of your learners.

The exercise sections begin with a section of topics that are mandated by the Joint Commission on the Accreditation of Healthcare Organizations (JCAHO) or others. Part 3 contains general teaching ideas that can be used in a variety of ways and adapted to your class flow and teaching plan. Part 4 addresses certain curriculum and continuing education topics. Advice from experience (Part 5) tells you what to expect when you use a new teaching approach.

The newest section is an index offered toward the end of the book. All the topics in the three *Instant Teaching Tools* series of books are indexed here so that you can see what other educators have used to teach the topics you are teaching. Check which volume each is located in before referencing the page number.

Variety of Learners

The methods contained in this book work with a wide variety of learners on both ends of the literacy scale. You can use these methods to teach volunteers, assistive personnel, students, and professional staff. The high involvement factor helps to overcome the gaps in age, experience, and culture. When asked to teach varied personnel and nontraditional learners in one group quickly, this book can serve as a valued resource. It also offers ideas you can use with one-to-one teaching.

This book is meant to be an easy reference and helpful tool to accomplish fun and creative educational offerings in health care facilities, schools of nursing, and allied health and training facilities of all kinds. Take some time to sample a few of these ideas. Select the ones you like best and try them. Try a new approach with some content that you know from past experience is hard to understand. You'll notice the difference in your learners and yourself. Remember, you have nothing to lose and everything to gain. Good luck and happy teaching!

PART 2
Instant Tools for Mandatories

Infection Control Crossword Puzzle

10 to 15 minutes   Laura Sumner, RN, Med, ONC

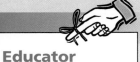

Tool box
- Infection control crossword puzzle
- Pens or pencils
- Answer key

Preparation

1. Make a copy of the ready-to-use Infection Control Crossword Puzzle for each participant.
2. Use this as introduction to the lesson, a review after the lesson, or as part of your required annual training.
3. Make sure all participants have a pen or pencil.
4. Make a copy of the answer key.

Implementation

1. Distribute the large or small crossword puzzle.
2. Challenge your learners to complete the puzzle as individuals or as teams.
3. If energy and attention are low during your lesson presentation, stop and let your participants engage in this energizing activity.
4. Crossword puzzles can act as pre- or posttests and can also be sent out days or weeks after the lesson to reinforce important concepts.

Variation

1. Use a poster printer copy machine to turn the crossword into a poster-sized image.
2. Plan for groups of two to six to discuss and fill in a poster-sized copy of the crossword puzzle before or after your lesson.

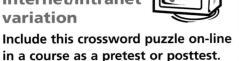

Educator secrets

If you have different ability levels in your session, pair learners to maximize benefits to all.

Internet/intranet variation

Include this crossword puzzle on-line in a course as a pretest or posttest.

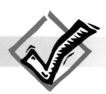

Infection Control Crossword Puzzle

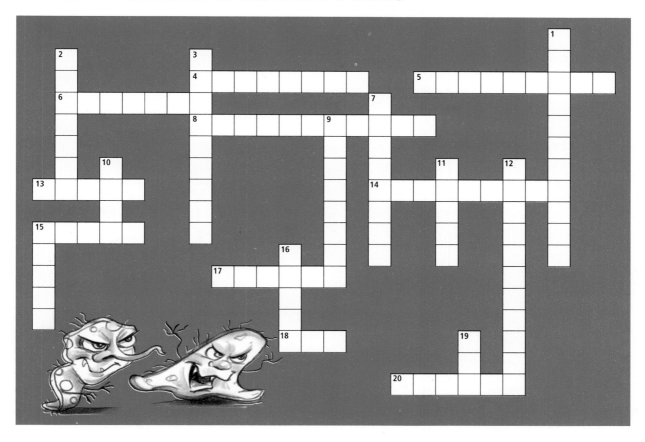

Across

4. _____ precautions are used for tuberculosis.
5. The two most common bloodborne pathogens are HIV and _____.
6. _____ precautions are used for MRSA, VRE, and C-diff.
8. _____ is the primary way to prevent the spread of disease.
13. _____ is a form of fungi.
14. MRSA and VRE are _____ to the usual antibiotics.
15. German measles, chickenpox, and cytomegalovirus are _____ infections that place unborn babies of nonimmune women at risk for congenital defects.
17. Tuberculosis is _____ through the air.
18. Infectious waste must be discarded into _____ -lined biohazard containers or red-lined waste buckets.
20. _____ are always worn when handling any blood or body fluids.

Down

1. Bacterial infections can be treated by _____.
2. A tiny organism seen by the microscope is called a _____.
3. _____ cause infection.
7. C-diff causes severe _____.
9. _____ precautions are used for everyone.
10. The regulatory agency that requires employers to ensure that health care workers use Standard Precautions with all patients is _____.
11. A _____ is the smallest microbe.
12. _____ are worn when there is a risk of body fluid splash, spray, or aerosol.
15. _____ is a disinfectant-detergent solution that is germicidal, fungicidal, and virucidal.
16. To prevent needle sticks _____ recap a needle.
19. Acquired immunodeficiency syndrome is caused by the _____ virus.

Infection Control Crossword Puzzle
ANSWER KEY

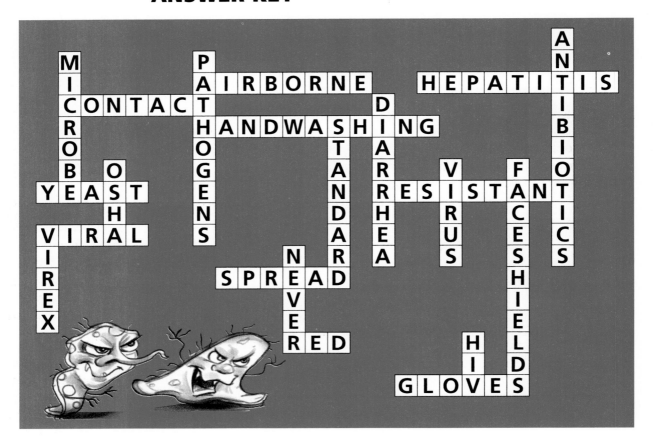

Across
4. Airborne
5. Hepatitis
6. Contact
8. Handwashing
13. Yeast
14. Resistant
15. Viral
17. Spread
18. Red
20. Gloves

Down
1. Antibiotics
2. Microbe
3. Pathogens
7. Diarrhea
9. Standard
10. OSHA
11. Virus
12. Faceshields
15. Virex
16. Never
19. HIV

Bag a Bug

Rhonda Scott-Foertsch, RN, BSN

Preparation

1. Make a list of common infectious organisms.
2. Prepare some information in each organism to add to the discussion.
3. Contact local institutions and compile some statistics (for class discussion) concerning the incidence of each organism.
4. Put together a resource center with the microbiology books, medical surgical nursing text, various laboratory slips, flip chart paper, and markers.

Implementation

1. Assign each person his or her own organism ("bug") from the list.
2. Give each person time to research the "bug."
3. Instruct each person to draw a picture of his or her "bug," telling them to make it fun and creative.
4. Have each person write a mini report on the organism including:
   a. What it is
   b. Where it is found
   c. What it can cause
5. Instruct each person to show and tell about his or her bug, including the picture and any lab slips that identify the organism.
6. Combine this activity with a class on infection control.

Tool box

- Flip chart paper
- Marking pens
- Microbiology books
- Lab slips
- Medical surgical nursing text
- *Optional:* Microscope and slides with organisms

Internet/intranet variation

In an on-line course, ask the participants to research each "bug" and post information on an on-line bulletin board.

Educator secrets

This is a good way to increase awareness about organisms in the health care environment.

5 to 10 minutes

The Story of Life

Michele L. Deck, RN, MEd, BSN, LCCE, FACCE

Tool box
- **Instructor's body language**

Preparation

1. Practice telling and acting out this story before you use it to teach a class.

Implementation

1. Say to your learners, "I have a story to tell you, but you must participate by repeating the word or words I point out to you."
2. Walk to a side wall of your classroom and pretend to shake it. Say, "I walk to the wall, and I *shake* it." As you move your arms have them repeat, "Shake."
3. Moving your arms in an arc toward the top of the wall continue with, "Large, red, neon letters appear on the wall that say *EMS*." As you move your arms have them repeat, "EMS" (emergency medical service).
4. Now repeat those two motions in order so that they repeat, "Shake" and "EMS."
5. Move your hand across the wall and say, "Now the wall has a jagged crack in it that runs from the top to the bottom, it is *open*. As you move your arms as if the wall is cracked, have them repeat, "Open."
6. Now repeat those three motions in order so that they repeat, "Shake, EMS, Open."
7. Open your hand, move it from left to right, and say, "In the opening of the wall stands a glove that looks like the Hamburger Helper mascot. It has eyes, nose, etc. Its name is Mr. *Look, Listen, Feel*." As you move your hand have them repeat, "Look, listen, feel."
8. Now repeat those four motions in order so that they repeat, "Shake, EMS, open, look, listen, feel."
9. Point to your right and say, "Imagine that Faith Hill, the singer, is behind a microphone here just finishing up the line of her song, *Just Breathe*. In fact, she has an identical twin who is singing an echo of her that says, *"Breathe."* Point to your right so that they repeat, "Breathe, breathe."

Educator secrets
Approach this with a sense of fun and drama.

16

10. Now repeat those five motions in order so that they repeat, "Shake, EMS, open, look, listen, feel, breathe, breathe."

11. Move to your right past the imaginary Faith Hill twins and hold both arms akimbo. Say, "There is a giant check mark watching the show here. There is a *check*." Have them repeat, "Check."

12. Now repeat those six motions in order so that they repeat, "Shake, EMS, open, look, listen, feel, breathe, breathe, check."

13. Explain, "The check begins to dance to the music and begins to *compress* 15 times until he is very tiny." Begin to slowly deflate downward as people say, "Compress, compress, compress, compress." Continue until the audience has said the word compress 15 times.

14. Now repeat those seven motions in order so that they repeat, "Shake, EMS, open, look, listen, feel, breathe, breathe, check, compress (15 times)."

15. Tell the group as soon as the check gets tiny, it springs back to full size. The Faiths repeat, "Breathe, breathe," and the check compresses again. This action loops on and on, or this action repeats.

16. Now repeat those seven motions in order so that they repeat, "Shake, EMS, open, look, listen, feel, breathe, breathe, check, compress (15 times), breathe, breathe, compress (15 times), breathe, breathe, compress (15 times), breathe, breathe."

17. Point to the door. Say, "Standing at the door is a single (one) Minute Man from history." Ask them who is there, and have them say, "One minute" as you point to the door.

18. Now repeat those eight motions in order so they repeat, "Shake, EMS, open, look, listen, feel, breathe, breathe, check, 1 minute."

19. Tell them the minute man yells, "Reassess."

20. Have them repeat, "Reassess."

21. Now point out to them that they know the steps to adult one-person cardiopulmonary resuscitation (CPR). Have them say the words while you or they demonstrate.
    a. **Shake** to determine unresponsiveness.
    b. Activate **EMS.**
    c. **Open** the airway.
    d. **Look, listen,** and **feel** for breathing.
    e. If not breathing, give **two breaths.**
    f. **Check** for a pulse.
    g. If no pulse, **compress 15 times** to every two breaths.
    h. Continue for **1 minute.**
    i. **Reassess.**

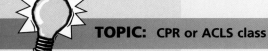

Who Do You Love Most in the World?

5 to 10 minutes for approximately 20 people in class

Donna McHenry, NREMT-P

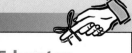

Tool box

- **Flipchart with markers, chalkboard with chalk, or whiteboard with markers**

Preparation

1. Draw three columns on the flipchart or chalkboard.
2. Label column one, "Name," column two, "Why" (for Why are you here?), and column three "Who"(for Who do you love most in the world?).
3. Ready a marker to use to record learner responses in each column.

Implementation

1. Introduce yourself to the class.
2. Go around the room and ask participants to introduce themselves by answering the three questions. Write each person's response under the appropriate column.
3. When everyone has answered, explain that during the class you want them to think about the person they have listed in column three and imagine that they collapse. Ask them to remain in class until they are confident that they would know exactly what to do if their loved one became their patient.
4. Assure them that you will stay as late as needed until they feel confident about their CPR or advanced cardiac life support ACLS skills.

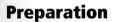

Educator secrets

Many people (even medical professionals) never think about the possibility of the victim being their loved one. When they do, everyone stays focused and the job of teaching is easier.

Your Deepest, Darkest Secret

Gina M. Ankner, MSN, RN, CS

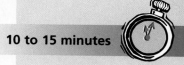

10 to 15 minutes

Preparation

1. Distribute an envelope, small index card, and pen or pencil to each participant.
2. Prepare one set for yourself.

Tool box
- **One envelope for yourself and one for each learner**
- **One index card for yourself and one for each learner**
- **Pen or pencil for yourself and each learner**

Implementation

1. Ask each participant to write on the index card something they have never told anyone; something that would embarrass them if a person in the room was to learn this about them—in other words, their deepest, darkest secret.
2. Agree to do this activity with the participants.
3. Once they have written something, each person seals the index card in the envelope.
4. Instruct them to pass their envelope to the person sitting on their right.
5. Ask the participants how do they feel now that another person has this information. How would they feel if the person holding their secret were to open the envelope and read their card? What if that person revealed their secret to others in the group?
6. Explain that health care professionals are allowed access to very private information about clients. This is information that even the client's own friends and family may not know. Clients trust health care professionals by virtue of what health care professionals represent and the confidentiality that is implied and expected from the profession.
7. Ask participants to consider the feelings they have regarding their secret being shared with the group and to remember this when they are in public places and tempted to discuss a client case or reveal confidential information.
8. Pass the envelopes back to their owners. How do they feel now, knowing their secret is safe?

Educator secrets
Participants are more likely to agree to this activity if the instructor models and participates as well. Although they may struggle at first, everyone can think of something to write on the index card that they would rather not reveal.

Prudent Living People Bingo

15 to 20 minutes Martin Isganitis, BS

Tool box
- **Prudent Living People Bingo Cards**
- **Pencil or pen for each learner**
- **Small prizes**

Preparation

1. Copy the different versions of Prudent Living People Bingo Card, one for each participant.
2. Distribute the Prudent Living People Bingo Cards and a pencil or pen to each learner.

Implementation

1. Announce the start of the game about 15 minutes before the class is scheduled to begin or when about one third of the participants have arrived.
2. Hold up a sample of the Prudent Living People Bingo Card and read the instructions.
3. Ask the learners to introduce themselves to other members of the class, one at a time.
4. Invite them to ask questions to find out which of the activities on the bingo card fits their life style.
5. Have each person place his or her initials in a square that fits his or her life style.
6. Clarify that each person may initial a bingo card in one square only per card.
7. The person may initial his or her own card in one space that fits his or her life style.
8. Explain that bingo is achieved when all of the spaces on the card are initialed.
9. Make it clear that each item on the Prudent Living People Bingo Card is an example of a behavior that can reduce the risk for heart disease and stroke. Ask the learners to identify the risk factors, to indicate which factors can be changed, and to explain which factors cannot be changed.

Educator secrets
People Bingo of any kind is a high-energy way to start any class. Instead of sitting quietly in their chairs, partici-pants are up and moving around the room, networking with others.

Internet/intranet variation

Include this bingo card on-line in a course, and ask learners to network with others to fill their paper copy of the bingo card.

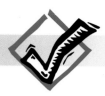

Prudent Living People Bingo Card

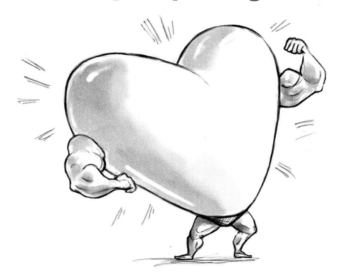

I generally avoid eating red meat.	I exercise moderately at least 30 minutes most days.	I remove and discard the skin from poultry before I cook and eat it.	I eat fewer than three egg yolks per week.
I use limited amounts of vegetable oils to prepare foods.	I recently reduced my cholesterol level through diet and exercise.	I maintain my optimal body weight.	I recently stopped smoking cigarettes.
I have never smoked cigarettes.	I eat broiled foods instead of fried foods.	I trim excess fat from red meats (beef, pork, lamb).	I know my cholesterol count.
I look for packaged foods suggested by the American Heart Association.	I know my normal blood pressure.	I eat foods low in salt and sodium.	I know which risk factors I have for heart disease.

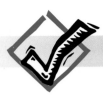

Prudent Living People Bingo Card

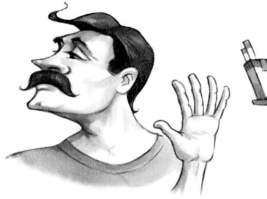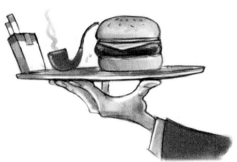

I know my cholesterol count.	I have never smoked cigarettes.	I generally avoid eating red meat.	I know my normal blood pressure.
I look for packaged foods suggested by the American Heart Association.	I know which risk factors I have for heart disease.	I remove and discard the skin from poultry before I cook and eat it.	I exercise moderately at least 30 minutes most days.
I eat fewer than three egg yolks per week.	I eat foods low in salt and sodium.	I recently stopped smoking cigarettes.	I eat broiled foods instead of fried foods.
I trim excess fat from red meats (beef, pork, lamb).	I maintain my optimal body weight.	I use limited amounts of vegetable oils to prepare foods.	I recently reduced my cholesterol level through diet and exercise.

Board Game Fun

Sherry Blanchard, RN

15 to 30 minutes

Preparation

1. Create one poster per policy or procedure to be learned or reviewed. (If you anticipate using the posters many times, laminate them.) Use local street names to identify each poster such as "Jones Avenue" or "Main Street." They also need to include six questions that learners can answer if they read the information on the poster. (Place questions at the bottom of the poster.)
2. Rotate each poster through break rooms and other highly visible areas of your facility.
3. Create a scorecard for participants to use, with one square for each policy and procedure poster listed on it. Make it appear like a game board around the outside of the card, naming each card to correspond to each poster.
4. Obtain a hole puncher for each host to use.
5. Once the posters have been rotated, select a room and time for all learners to review all of them in anticipation of Joint Commission or some other yearly mandate.
6. Place four 8-foot long tables end to end to form a rectangle.
7. Position your volunteer game hosts in the center of the tables that form a rectangle.
8. Place the posters side by side to form a giant game board. Place an asterisk (*) next to five out of all of the questions on all of the boards.
9. Ready the prizes.
10. Distribute one die and one hole puncher to each game host.
11. Position the box for the larger prize drawing at the door to the room.

Continued

Tool box
- Four 8-foot long tables
- Large dice, as many as hosts
- Scorecard game cards for punching
- One hole puncher per game host
- One poster per policy or procedure to be learned or reviewed
- Small prizes
- One larger prize
- Recruited participants to act as game hosts
- One box for scorecard drawing

Educator secrets
You can assign people to groups and have them work together as a team to complete one scorecard for all. This idea is a great way to ready a facility for a Joint Commission review.

Board Game Fun—cont'd

Implementation

1. Distribute a scorecard to each learner.
2. Ask the participant to begin anywhere on the board by selecting a policy or procedure, street or deed.
3. A host hands them the big die and they roll it.
4. Whichever number comes up on the die is the question that he or she must answer on that poster board (if a 6 is rolled, he or she must answer question 6).
5. Participants can use the reference material on the poster to answer.
6. To make it more exciting, if the number he or she rolled was one of the preselected winning numbers (marked by an asterisk [*]), a small prize is awarded to the learner.
7. After answering the question correctly, the host punches a hole in the scorecard and moves with that person to another game piece. Play continues until the learners have answered a question at every game piece and have a punched hole for every square on the scorecard.
8. The learner then places his or her name on the completed card and places it in a box so that it is entered in a drawing for a bigger prize.

Emergency Response Questions, Not Answers

Iris Trahan, RN, BSN, CCRN

15 to 30 minutes

Tool box
- **Game board with categories and point amounts on overhead transparency (projector), PowerPoint screens (computer and display setup), or posters**
- **Answer sheets**
- **Question sheet**
- **Buzzing device**
- **Self-adhesive notes**
- **Watch with a second hand or timing device**
- **Variety of small prizes**

Preparation

1. Review the information on the ready-to-use answer sheet and questions sheet, and make any adaptations necessary to your facility.
2. Create a projectable image of the amount and category sheet. (An overhead transparency or PowerPoint screen is best, but a poster will also work.)
3. Copy the answer sheet for yourself. This is for you to read to the learners when they pick a category and an amount.
4. Make a copy of the Answer Key questions (for you to check your learners' responses).
5. Obtain a buzzing device to determine which team rings in first.
6. Place self-adhesive notes on the category and amount transparency or poster squares after they have been chosen. Place an X over PowerPoint squares. This will make it easy for the learners to see what can still be chosen.
7. Collect a variety of small prizes or goodies (fruit, stickers, pins, pens, etc.) to award to participants at the end of the activity.

Implementation

1. Divide the group into two or more teams of three to six learners.
2. Explain that the teams may collaborate before answering the question.
3. Present the categories:
   a. "Just Say No" has to do with code medications.
   b. Shock/Shock/Shock is focused on defibrillation.
   c. Blues Clues is respiratory information.
   d. Pacing is about itself, that is, pacing.

Educator secrets
Create a fun atmosphere and equalize participation as much as possible.

Continued

Emergency Response Questions,
Not Answers—cont'd

4. Select a team to go first. Display the playing board. A spokesperson for the group selects a category and an amount.
5. The instructor reads the answer from that category and the amount.
6. The teams can discuss their ideas quietly for up to 5 seconds before answering.
7. A team representative states the question that fits the answer the instructor has given.
8. If the question given is correct, the team is awarded points based on how much their question was worth. If the answer is incorrect, the instructor can give the other teams a chance to answer or simply reveal the correct answer. If the question has an asterisk (*) by it, the team can wager as many points as they might have.
9. Points are tallied for each team.
10. After all answers are given, the team with the most points wins.
11. Prizes are awarded to all participants, with those with the highest points selecting their gifts first. Because their knowledge has increased, they are all winners.

Internet/intranet variation
This can be used as a pretest or posttest or review in an Internet course.

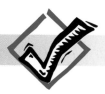

Emergency Response Questions, Not Answers
AMOUNT AND CATEGORY SHEET

DIRECTIONS: This playing board can be made into a projectable visual or a poster.

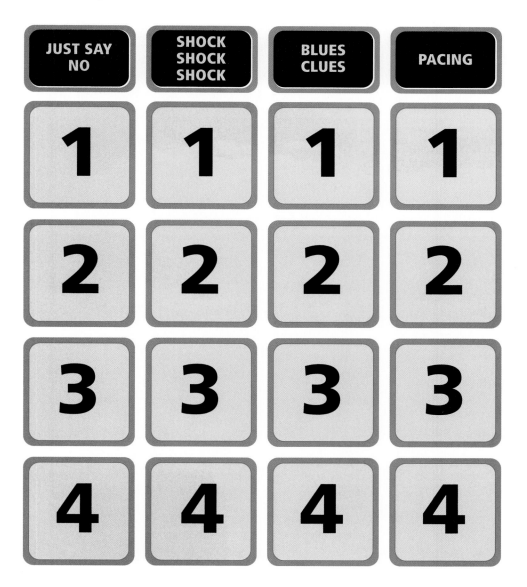

Emergency Response Questions, Not Answers
ANSWERS

DIRECTIONS: This playing board can be made into an overhead transparency or downloaded into power point.

JUST SAY NO	SHOCK SHOCK SHOCK	BLUES CLUES	PACING
After oxygen, this is the first code drug used in VF.	Defibrillation is used for this dysrhythmia.	This drug is used to treat hypoxia.	This device can externally pace the patient.
This drug is used for symptomatic bradycardia.	This chant is used to clear bystanders and staff before defibrillation.	Name for difficult or labored breathing.	TCP would be used for this rhythm.
This drug used for SVT is given in a rapid bolus.	Synchronized shock used in unstable SVT or other unstable supraventricular rhythms.	The rate of rescue breathing in the adult apneic patient.	Setting on the TCP that regulates the amount of energy the machine puts forth for pacing.
This drug in the dose of 300 mg is given in VF.	Sequence of energy levels used for VF with a monoplastic defibrillator in the adult patient.	Device that assesses the endotracheal tube placement by changing from purple to yellow.	Name that represents that each pacer output results in an ECG complex.

VF, Ventricular fibrillation, *TCP, transcutaneous pacemaker; SVT, supraventricular tachycardia; ECG, electrocardiographic.*

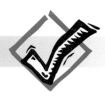

Emergency Response Questions, Not Answers
ANSWERS KEY QUESTIONS

DIRECTIONS: This playing board can be made into an overhead transparency, downloaded into PowerPoint, or used as your answer key copied on paper. The learner should place his or her answer in the form of a question, as shown following.

JUST SAY NO	SHOCK SHOCK SHOCK	BLUES CLUES	PACING
What is epinephrine?	What is VF or pulseless VT?	What is oxygen?	What is TCP?
What is atropine?	What is "I'm going to shock on three. One, I'm clear. Two, you're clear. Three, we're all clear?"	What is dyspnea?	What is symptomatic bradycardia?
What is adenosine or adenocard?	What is synchronized or electrical cardioversion?	What is 12/minute?	What is MA?
What is aminodarone?	What is 200 J, 200 to 300 J, 300 J?	What is an end-tidal CO_2 detector?	What is capture?

5 to 7 minutes

Brush with Fame

Michele L. Deck, RN, MEd, BSN, LCCE, FACCE

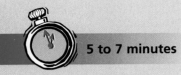

Tool box
No tools are needed.

Preparation

1. Think about which "brush with fame" story you will tell the group.
2. It is important that you model this activity.

Implementation

1. At the beginning of class, divide your attendees into teams of three to six members.
2. Select a leader of each team in a fun way (such as who owns the largest pet).
3. Explain that each person has to think back into their memory of when they have had a "brush with fame" in their personal life. Have they ever seen someone with a recognizable name live and in person? It could be some local or national celebrity. For example, it could be a local politician or newscaster, a singer, an actor, a musician, or an athlete. Have they ever attended a live performance of someone famous or just run into someone on the street? Each person will get to share his or her story with the rest of the team after you tell yours.
4. Relate your brush with fame.
5. Announce the group leader is responsible for making sure each team member gets to tell his or her story. Offer the teams a 5-minute time limit to finish all stories.
6. Tell the group when time has expired.

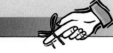

Educator secrets
Learners who have worked together for many years may be surprised when their coworkers relate these stories, because they may not have heard them before. This works well with groups that know each other and groups that do not.

Internet/intranet variation
Ask learners in your on-line course to post their "brush with fame" on an electronic bulletin board. This helps people to make a human connection with others who may only be a screen name before this activity. It offers something to make each person unique and memorable.

7. Sometimes a group demands that one team member relate his or her story to the group, because it is just too good to miss. Invite that person to tell the story to the entire group.
8. You can then highlight the difference between one's personal and professional life. If we encounter famous people when we are working in a professional role, we cannot tell that to anyone. Highlight the importance of privacy, confidentiality, and new Health Insurance Portability and Accountability (HIPAA) standards.

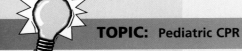

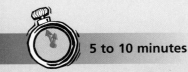 **TOPIC:** Pediatric CPR

 5 to 10 minutes

String Along

Michele L. Deck, RN, MEd, BSN, LCCE, FACCE

Preparation

1. Copy the String Along ready-to-use pages.
2. Copy the answer key.
3. Place the string and scissors close to you.

Implementation

1. Recruit nine volunteers to come up to the front and each hold one part (written on the ready-to-use pages) of the process used to perform CPR on a child aged 1 to 8 years.
2. Ask the volunteers to randomly select one of the ready-to-use pages and stand in a half circle, so the rest of the class can see their signs.
3. Hand the string to the person holding the "Determine unresponsiveness" paper. Announce this is the first step in performing CPR on a child.
4. Holding onto the end of the string, this person passes the string to the person holding the sign that says "Call for help," no matter where he or she is standing.
5. The person holding the sign that says "Call for help" now holds the middle portion of the string he or she received and passes the ball of string onto the person holding the sign that says "Open the airway."
6. The person holding the sign that says "Open the airway" holds onto the middle portion of the string and passes the ball of string to the person holding the sign that says "Look, listen, and feel for breathing."
7. This process continues until all the participants are holding onto a piece of the string and the person holding the sign that says "After 1 minute if no response and alone, activate EMS" has the rest of the ball of string.
8. Emphasize to the group the importance and interrelationship of all the steps.
9. Use the scissors to snip any one piece of string between two of the steps. Ask the learners what would happen if the sequence of CPR for a child were to stop at that point.
10. Foster a discussion of what to do in a crisis (represented by the cut made by the scissors) and how to continue through the steps to achieve the best possible outcome for the patient.

Tool box
- **Ball of string**
- **Scissors**
- **String Along ready-to-use pages**
- **String Along answer key**

Educator secrets
Cutting the string serves as a way to make the consequences of inaction tangible to learners.

32

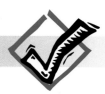

String Along Card

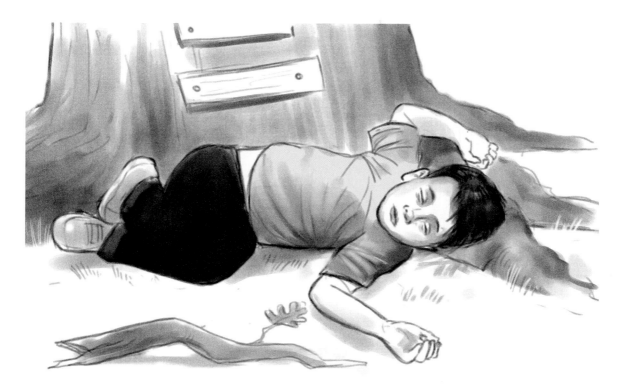

Determine unresponsiveness.

String Along Card

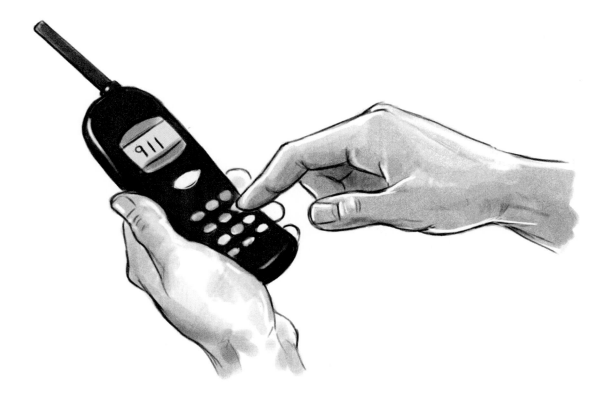

Call for help.
Direct someone to call EMS.

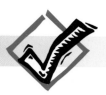

String Along Card

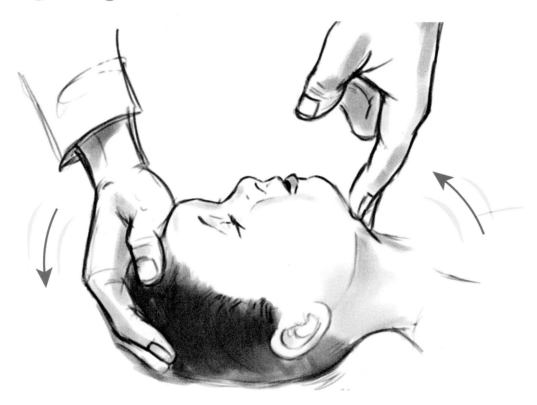

Open the airway.

String Along Card

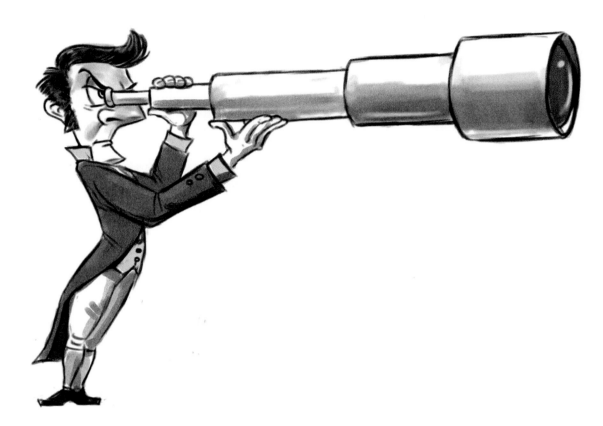

Look, listen, and feel for breathing.

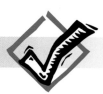

String Along Card

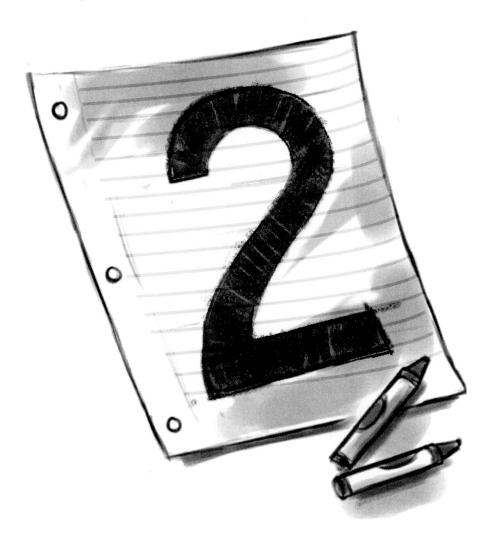

No breathing.
Give two breaths.

String Along Card

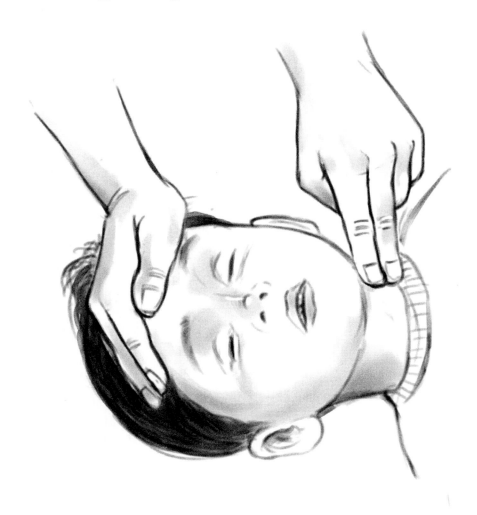

Check for a carotid pulse.

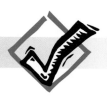

String Along Card

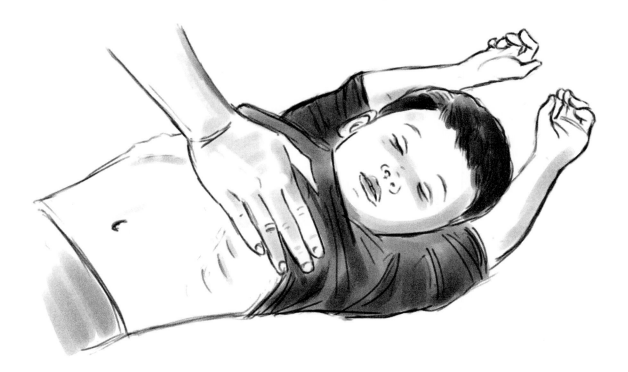

No pulse. Compress chest 100 times per minute.

String Along Card

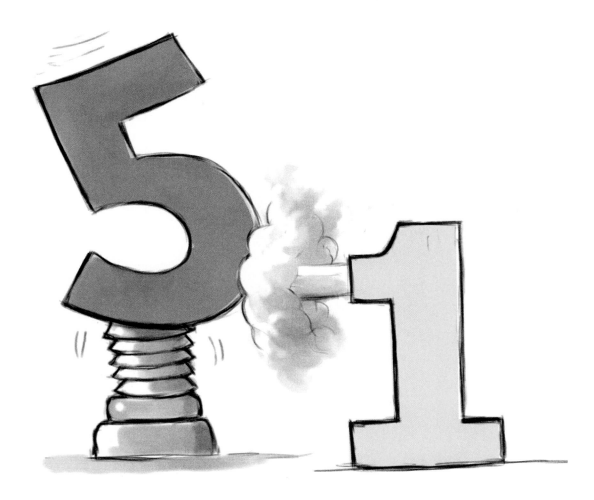

Give one breath after every five compressions.

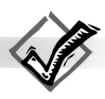

String Along Card

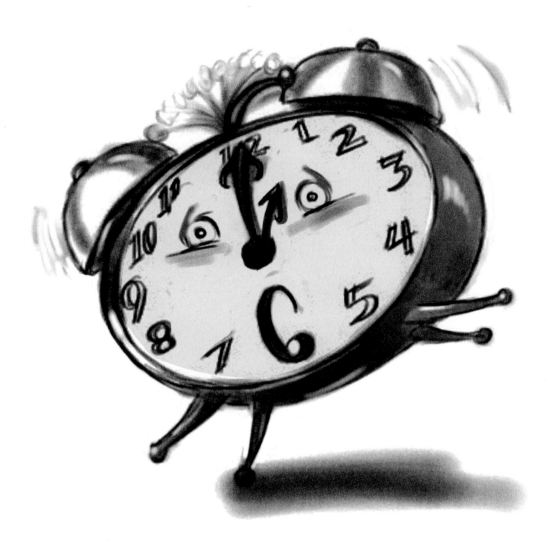

If no response after 1 minute and alone, activate EMS.

String Along Card
ANSWER KEY

Determine unresponsiveness.
Call for help. Direct someone to call EMS.
Open the airway.
Look, listen, and feel for breathing.
No breathing. Give two breaths.
Check for a carotid pulse.
No pulse. Compress 100 times per minute.
Give one breath after every five compressions
If no response after 1 minute and alone, activate EMS.

Don't Use This If...

Michele L. Deck, RN, MEd, BSN, LCCE, FACCE

5 minutes

Preparation

1. Practice drawing the simple pictures in the grid.
2. Distribute an index card to each learner.

Implementation

1. Draw a blank grid on your acetate or flipchart page.
2. In the top left-hand corner, draw the picture, keeping it as simple as possible. Explain how this represents never using an automated external defibrillator (AED) on a child under the age of 8 years old.
3. Draw the picture in the top right of the box. Explain how this represents that a victim in water should not be attached to an AED.
4. Draw the picture in the bottom left corner of the grid. Tell the group how this picture represents the fact that someone with a pacemaker or internal defibrillator is not a candidate for use of an AED.
5. Draw the picture on the bottom right. This represents the fact that a person wearing a medication patch should not be hooked to an AED until the patch is removed and the drug wiped off the area.
6. Point to each box and ask the learners to verbally tell you what the pictures represent.
7. Draw a blank grid. Point to each of the boxes and ask what picture appeared in the box.
8. Invite all learners to create the blank grid on their index cards.
9. Ask the learners to draw in the pictures from memory.
10. Invite the learners to slip the index cards into their pockets to take home and use if they are faced with using an AED.

Tool box
- **Don't Use This If...ready-to-use pictures for drawing**
- **One index card per learner**
- **Overhead projector with a blank piece of acetate or a flipchart with markers**

Educator secrets
Keep the pictures very simple so that all participants can copy and remember them easily.

Don't Use This If...Pictures

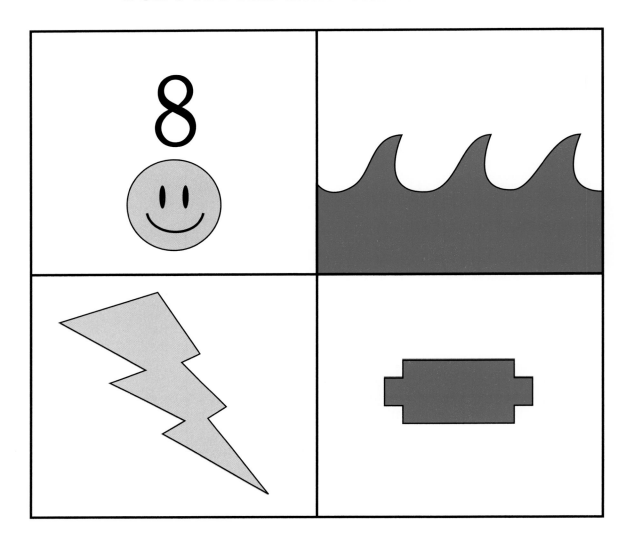

Fact or Fiction

Michele L. Deck, RN, MEd, BSN, LCCE, FACCE

5 minutes

Preparation

1. Make the facts into a visual.
2. Project it before the group.

Implementation

1. Explain to the group that three of the facts are true and one is false. Can they detect the false fact?
2. Ask the learners to vote by show of hands which is the false fact. Ask them for their reasons.
3. Reveal the false fact.
4. Foster a discussion on the facts and fiction.

Educator secrets
You can personalize this activity to any content you have. Select hard facts for use.

Internet/intranet variation
Have learners vote on bulletin board areas as to which fact they think is false and why.

Fact or Fiction

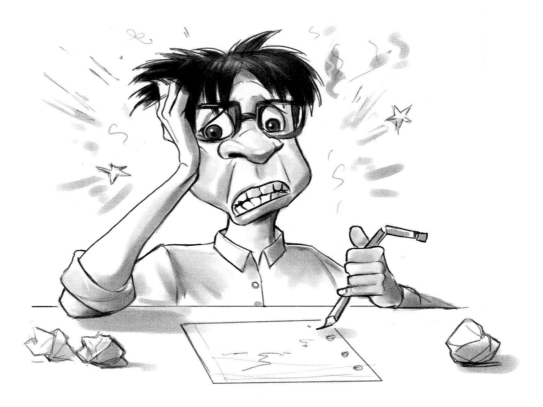

1. The majority of the population of the United States is over 35 years of age.
2. Heart disease is the number one chronic disease in the United States.
3. An AED can be used on a patient wearing a medication patch if you remove it first and wipe the area.
4. Eye protection and gloves should be used when performing CPR.

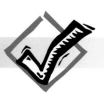

Fact or Fiction
ANSWER KEY

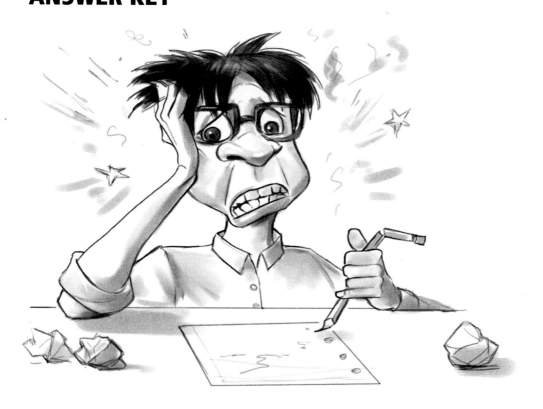

1. The majority of the population of the United States is over 35 years of age.
   True, according to data from the U.S. Census in 2003.
2. Heart disease is the number one chronic disease in the United States by occurrence.
   False, according to the TeleNation for Novaris Pharmaceutical Corporation. In 2003, irritable bowel syndrome (IBS) topped the list at 40 million, followed by depression at 19 million, asthma and diabetes at 17 million, and heart disease at 12.5 million.
3. An AED can be used on a patient wearing a medication patch if you remove it and wipe the area first.
   True, according to the American Heart Association.
4. Eye protection and gloves should be used when performing CPR.
   True, according to the American Heart Association. One should also use a mask or barrier for breathing.

TOPIC: Annual Reviews: Customer service, operating room information, nursing process, crash cart, specimen information, blood transfusions, fire safety

Approximately 30 minutes, depending on the number of teams and amount of follow-up discussion

Building Knowledge Bottom to Top

Jennifer Kadis, MSN, RN, CPAN
JoAnn Segarra, RN, BSN, CNOR

Preparation

1. Copy the ready-to-use RN or Surgical Technician Knowledge sheet on an overhead sheet or download into PowerPoint. Cover each category with a Post-It note (or some other small cover) when using an overhead projector, or display only one category at a time on PowerPoint.
2. Provide two chairs (facing each other, in the front of the room) with a good view of the screen.
3. Decide on the point value for each category. Generally, simpler items are placed along the bottom and are worth fewer points. The hardest (or most important) category is placed at the top and is worth the most points.

Implementation

1. Select two players. If using teams, ask each team to select two players. Send the players outside the room and bring them in one team at a time, so they cannot see or hear the clues.
2. Set a timer for 5 minutes.

Tool box
- Overhead projector or PowerPoint (with computer and projector)
- Game format on an overhead or computer screen
- Two single chairs (facing each other) just in front of the overhead machine
- Timing device or stopwatch
- Small prizes

Internet/intranet variation

Post in on-line course and have learners list the clues under the categories to determine comprehension of procedures.

3. One player, the "talker," will sit facing the information; the other player, the "guesser," will sit facing the talker so that he or she cannot see the screen. The instructor will display one category at a time, and the talker provides descriptive clues until the guesser correctly names the category. The talker may not use any of the same words that are in the category. For example, if the category is "Things needed to start an IV," the talker may say things like "a tubing, a catheter, a dressing," but he or she cannot say the word "IV" or that category is forfeited.

4. Any category may be "put on hold" and returned to at the end, time permitting.

5. Team members may cheer or encourage but may not give clues.

6. The team with the most points wins the game.

7. Distribute small prizes.

Educator secrets

You may have to give a demonstration before the game begins, particularly with younger learners or those from another country. When the game is finished, review any categories that any team had difficulty with or ask each team to talk about the high points of a given category.

Building Knowledge Bottom to Top
RN KNOWLEDGE

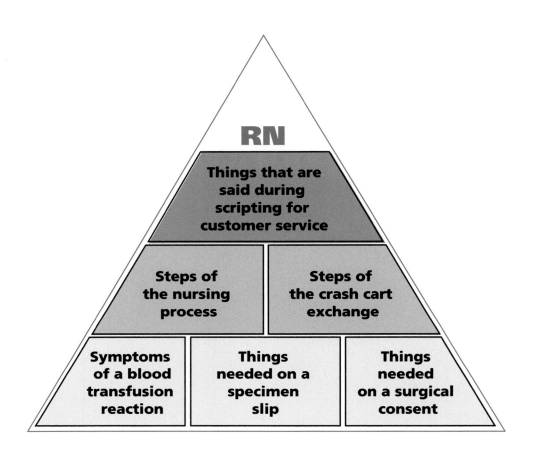

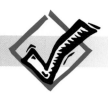

Building Knowledge Bottom to Top
SURGICAL TECHNICIAN KNOWLEDGE

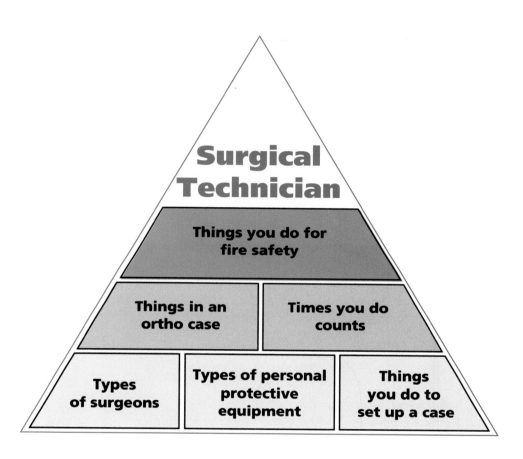

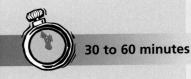

Surgical Services Emergency Relay

Jennifer Kadis, MSN, RN, CPAN
JoAnn Segarra, RN, BSN, CNOR

30 to 60 minutes

Tool box
- **One baton for each team**
- **One touch light or bell for each team to activate when their team is finished**
- **One list of tasks per team—see handout (If one team has less members, some members may have to go twice.)**
- **Small prizes**
- **All necessary equipment (you can adjust this to fit your needs, but try to ensure that performance of each task requires about the same amount of time):**
  - **Adult crash cart**
  - **Pediatric crash cart**
  - **Pediatric manikin**
  - **Broselow tape**
  - **Malignant hyperthermia cart**
  - **Defibrillator with pacing capability**

Preparation

1. Line the teams up next to each other at one end of the room. Team members should be single file and are not allowed to look at their assigned task until the team member directly in front of them passes it to them.
2. Space the equipment around the room. The task sheets are designed so that no teams go to the same piece of equipment at the same time (to provide enough room to work). If possible, position a spotter at each piece of equipment to ensure the task is fully and correctly completed.
3. Tear the tasks sheets into individual strips. Each team gets only their own tasks, and all tasks must be done in order.

Educator secrets
This is a high-energy activity and works well after lunch or after a long lecture. If all participants are very familiar with the equipment, change the tasks to locating low-usage items. Try to arrange the groups so that skill levels are approximately equal (e.g., not all pediatric nurses on the same team). At the end of the game it will be readily apparent to each participant where his or her personal deficiencies are, usually without much input from the instructor. Ask participants to share their frustrations regarding what they could not locate or operate quickly. Relate this exercise to having to perform quickly in an emergency and the need to stay familiar with all the emergency equipment—this is the most important part of the activity!

Implementation

1. Give the first person in line the task sheet and the baton. He or she performs the first task on the sheet and then comes back to the line and hands off the baton to the second person in line. That person performs the second task and hands off to the third person and so on (so that team members cannot see their tasks ahead of time).

2. The first team to complete all tasks wins. Although the team may not give members instruction on how to complete a task, cheering and team support is encouraged.

3. The game continues until all teams have finished. When the game is finished, break up into groups to review the carts and equipment in depth.

4. Distribute prizes.

Surgical Services Emergency Relay

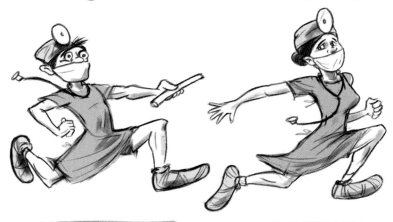

	TEAM 1	TEAM 2	TEAM 3	TEAM 4
1	**Defibrillation**	**Code Cart**	**MH Cart**	**Pediatric Cart**
	Set defibrillator to 220 J and correct	Adenocard 5 cc syringe and needle	Mannitol	Measure baby and pull correct color bag
2	**Pediatric Cart**	**Defibrillation**	**Code Cart**	**MH Cart**
	Ambu the baby	Set defibrillator to 360 J and shock	Dopamine drip and tubing	Lasix
3	**MH Cart**	**Pediatric Cart**	**Defibrillation**	**Code Cart**
	Find the dantrolene	Measure baby and pull correct color bag	Set pacer to 70 J and pace	No. 7 endotracheal tube, stylet, and laryngoscope
4	**Code Cart**	**MH Cart**	**Pediatric Cart**	**Defibrillation**
	Epinephrine	Sterile water and transfer set	Atropine	Set defibrillator to synchronize shock at 200 J and shock
5	**Defibrillation**	**Code Cart**	**MH Cart**	**Pediatric Cart**
	Set pacer at 80 J, correct, and pace	Nasogastric tube and 30 cc syringe	Blood gas kit	Measure baby and pull correct color bag
6	**Pediatric Cart**	**Defibrillation**	**Code Cart**	**MH Cart**
	Lidocaine	Set defibrillator to 300 J and shock	Lidocaine drip and tubing	CVP kit

MH, Malignant hyperthermia; *CVP,* central venous pressure.

PART 3
Instant Tools
for Learning Ideas

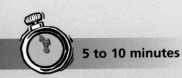
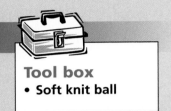

5 to 10 minutes

Bouncing Around

Susan Bosold, MS, MA, RN

Tool box
- **Soft knit ball**

Preparation

1. Ask your participants to sit in chairs.
2. Obtain soft ball.

Implementation

1. Explain that the object of the activity is to see how many tosses they can accomplish as a group without dropping the ball. They must toss it to someone who is at least six seats away from them in either direction.
2. Each person can only receive the ball once. (If someone has already caught it, he or she can't catch it again during the current round.)
3. Keep track and only count it when they make an improvement. (If someone had six successful tosses the previous round, he or she must get at least seven during the current round.)
4. Toss the ball to someone.
5. The whole audience counts, "One, two, three, four, five..."
6. The performance has to exceed the previous highest number to count. If it does, they get an extra 3 minutes at break or some pre-determined reward.

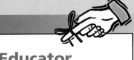

Educator secrets
This promotes concentration, support, and the whole group working for the good of all.

These Hands of Mine

Vivian Jefferson, RN, MSN

Preparation

1. Distribute worksheet and pens or pencils to each participant.

Implementation

1. Ask each person to write his or her first name in the box using the nondominant hand.
2. When they are finished writing their names, ask them to answer the five questions below the box on the worksheet.
3. Compare the feeling of learning a new skill to writing with the nondominant hand.
4. Facilitate a discussion on change and how uncomfortable, odd, and difficult it may feel at first, much like writing with the nondominant hand.

Tool box
- One pen for each learner
- One pencil for each learner
- One "Hands of Mine" worksheet for each learner

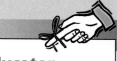

Educator secrets
Approach this in a fun and light-hearted way.

These Hands of Mine Worksheet

DIRECTIONS: Write your first name in the box using your nondominant hand.

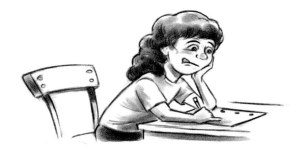

1. What knowledge did you have before you attempted this exercise?

2. How much previous experience did you have?

3. Did you feel competent writing your name in the past?

4. How did you feel?

5. Did it take you longer?

Question Query

Mary LaBiche, MEd, RRT

10 to 15 minutes

Preparation

1. Create one to three or more questions at different cognitive levels on the appropriate topic.
2. Try to use at least one analytical question.

Implementation

1. Hand out the questions to the students or put them on an overhead or PowerPoint presentation.
2. Ask the students to answer the questions.
3. After they have answered the questions, go over the answers and the type of question (recall, application, or analysis).
4. Review the thought processes and application of the material needed to answer the question correctly.

Tool box
- Written questions on a topic you are currently teaching. (Write questions on a topic of which you are currently teaching. Bring a few questions to class on different cognitive levels, such as recall, application, and analysis.)

Educator secrets
Have you ever heard a learner say, "The questions on the test were so much harder than the ones we went over in class."? This helps the instructor teach at a higher level and not just test at that level. It also helps the students to learn how to think analytically using the information presented. Health care educators need to focus on ways to help students to think critically.

15 to 30 minutes throughout entire class day

How May I Serve You?

Cheryl Burnette, MEd, RN

Tool box
- **Essential oils in a spray with sterile water (You might use lavender, a citrus scent, or both.)**
- **Small table**
- **Massage chair or hand or foot massagers**
- **Comfortable chair**
- **Crown (optional)**
- **Vase of flowers (optional)**

Preparation

1. Set up the massage chair with a small table beside it.
2. Put the essential oil spray on the table.
3. Add a vase of flowers to the table as well, if you would like to do so.
4. Include a crown for the participants to wear, if they desire to do so.

Implementation

1. At the beginning of a full class day, set out the "Throne" (i.e., chair) and all the items on the table.
2. Explain to the group that using available resources is very important. The massage chair is a resource available for any of the participants to use throughout the whole day.
3. Ask for a volunteer and demonstrate the use of the chair, including the settings.
4. When each volunteer is finished, encourage him or her to seek out another class member to use the chair.
5. The person who leaves the chair helps the new person to the chair by bringing items he or she may need to continue in class, such as his or her notebook or beverage.
6. Ask the person to review the workings of the chair with the new user. This encourages helping and supportive behavior among the participants.

Educator secrets
The chair is usually running most of the day, and participants will ask how to purchase one for their use. Participants say they are more relaxed and comfortable, so this can enhance learning. This is of particular importance in an organization that wants staff to use stress management strategies and resources.

Modeling and Role Modeling Word Search

Sandy Wilbanks, RN, BSN, CDE

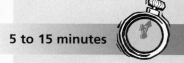

Preparation

1. Make a copy of the ready-to-use Modeling and Role Modeling Word Search Puzzle for each participant.
2. Use this as introduction to the lesson or review after the lesson.
3. Make sure all participants have a pen or pencil.
4. Make a copy of the answer key.

Tool box
- **Modeling and Role Modeling Word Search**
- **One pen or pencil per learner**

Variation

1. Use a poster printer copy machine to turn the word search puzzle into a poster-sized image.
2. Plan for groups of two to six to discuss and fill in a poster-sized copy of the puzzle before or after your lesson.

Implementation

1. Distribute the large or small Modeling and Role Modeling Word Search.
2. Challenge your learners to complete the puzzle as individuals or as teams.
3. If energy and attention are low during your lesson presentation, stop and let your participants engage in this energizing activity.
4. Word search puzzles can act as pre- or posttests and can also be sent out days or weeks after the lesson as reinforcement of important concepts.

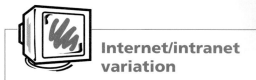

Internet/intranet variation

Include this word search puzzle on-line in a course as a review opportunity.

Educator secrets

If you have different ability levels in your session, pair learners to maximize benefits to all.

Modeling and Role Modeling Word Search

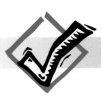
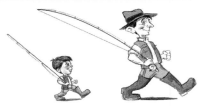

NAME															
ABILITY	H	L	M	U	O	P	E	R	H	P	T	A	S	K	P
ACCEPTANCE	I	K	D	B	H	I	M	S	O	S	R	K	T	F	O
ADAPTATION	N	A	G	E	V	B	S	E	L	F	C	A	R	E	I
AGE	A	D	S	C	F	E	E	L	I	N	G	S	E	F	N
ALIKE, APAM	M	A	B	I	L	I	T	Y	S	I	K	G	S	N	T
CARE	M	P	A	R	A	D	I	G	M	U	D	C	S	K	E
COPE	H	T	I	O	R	V	L	O	N	J	R	O	N	S	R
CONCEPT	D	A	G	L	C	P	U	A	P	A	M	N	P	T	V
COPING (2)	E	T	O	E	C	H	U	L	M	H	K	C	A	R	E
DATA	D	I	L	M	O	D	E	L	I	N	G	E	S	E	N
DIFFERENT	K	O	O	O	P	M	O	L	I	F	B	P	E	S	T
EMPATHY	Y	N	X	D	I	F	F	E	R	E	N	T	R	S	I
ENABLE	S	S	X	E	N	M	O	N	E	E	G	H	I	O	O
FEELINGS	W	A	Q	L	G	H	D	A	D	Y	V	B	S	R	N
GOAL	R	A	L	I	K	E	H	B	R	T	A	S	K	S	S
HEALTH	F	C	D	N	C	A	C	L	N	R	W	E	S	S	C
HOLISM	Y	C	O	G	L	L	N	E	N	U	N	C	O	P	E
HOPE	T	E	G	D	A	T	A	M	J	S	E	U	X	A	B
INTERVENTIONS	F	P	N	F	G	H	O	P	E	T	D	R	J	T	M
MODELING	S	T	A	G	E	S	U	A	B	H	S	E	T	I	N
PARADIGM	W	A	D	M	H	J	N	T	R	U	T	H	E	E	X
PATIENT	N	N	K	L	M	H	T	H	G	T	A	N	M	N	N
ROLE MODELING	C	C	O	P	I	N	G	Y	V	Y	G	N	L	T	B
SELF CARE	Z	E	E	Q	S	E	D	F	B	H	E	L	M	H	G
SECURE	C	D	G	N	L	O	I	Y	J	R	S	C	S	B	N
STAGES (2), STRESS	F	H	J	M	N	B	T	R	E	W	S	D	C	X	Z
STRESSORS, TASK (2)	U	M	P	O	J	N	G	H	Y	T	R	E	S	D	C
TRUST, TRUTH	H	B	F	R	E	D	S	W	E	A	X	Z	N	L	I

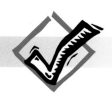

Modeling and Role Modeling Word Search
ANSWER KEY

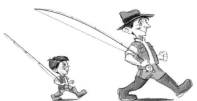

NAME														
ABILITY	H	L	M	U	O	P	E	R	H	P	T	A	S	K	P
ACCEPTANCE	I	K	D	B	H	I	M	S	O	S	R	K	T	F	O
ADAPTATION	N	A	G	E	V	B	S	E	L	F	C	A	R	E	I
AGE	A	D	S	C	F	E	E	L	I	N	G	S	E	F	N
ALIKE, APAM	M	A	B	I	L	I	T	Y	S	I	K	G	S	N	T
CARE	M	P	A	R	A	D	I	G	M	U	D	C	S	K	E
COPE	H	T	I	O	R	V	L	O	N	J	R	O	N	S	R
CONCEPT	D	A	G	L	C	P	U	A	P	A	M	N	P	T	V
COPING (2)	E	T	O	E	C	H	U	L	M	H	K	C	A	R	E
DATA	D	I	L	M	O	D	E	L	I	N	G	E	S	E	N
DIFFERENT	K	O	O	O	P	M	O	L	I	F	B	P	E	S	T
EMPATHY	Y	N	X	D	I	F	F	E	R	E	N	T	R	S	I
ENABLE	S	S	X	E	N	M	O	N	E	E	G	H	I	O	O
FEELINGS	W	A	Q	L	G	H	D	A	D	Y	V	B	S	R	N
GOAL	R	A	L	I	K	E	H	B	R	T	A	S	K	S	S
HEALTH	F	C	D	N	C	A	C	L	N	R	W	E	S	S	C
HOLISM	Y	C	O	G	L	L	N	E	N	U	N	C	O	P	E
HOPE	T	E	G	D	A	T	A	M	J	S	E	U	X	A	B
INTERVENTIONS	F	P	N	F	G	H	O	P	E	T	D	R	J	T	M
MODELING	S	T	A	G	E	S	U	A	B	H	S	E	T	I	N
PARADIGM	W	A	D	M	H	J	N	T	R	U	T	H	E	E	X
PATIENT	N	N	K	L	M	H	T	H	G	T	A	N	M	N	N
ROLE MODELING	C	C	O	P	I	N	G	Y	V	Y	G	N	L	T	B
SELF CARE	Z	E	E	Q	S	E	D	F	B	H	E	L	M	H	G
SECURE	C	D	G	N	L	O	I	Y	J	R	S	C	S	B	N
STAGES (2), STRESS	F	H	J	M	N	B	T	R	E	W	S	D	C	X	Z
STRESSORS, TASK (2)	U	M	P	O	J	N	G	H	Y	T	R	E	S	D	C
TRUST, TRUTH	H	B	F	R	E	D	S	W	E	A	X	Z	N	L	I

TOPIC: Communication, listening skills, focusing on others

Take the Communication Challenge

15 to 20 minutes

Sandra Stokes, RN

Tool box

- **Three clothespins per learner**
- **A few small prizes from which to choose**
- **Take the Communication Challenge Questionnaire**

Preparation

1. Copy the Take the Communication Challenge questionnaire, one per person.
2. Distribute three clothespins to each participant.
3. Ask each learner to pin them on his or her clothes or hold them in his or her hand.

Implementation

1. Explain to everyone that the purpose of this activity is to get the other person to talk to you about himself by asking and answering questions.
2. Say, "You now have an opportunity to learn about each other. You will not be asked to share specific statements made by each other while you participate in this activity. Listening is critical to good communication, and the good listener focuses on what the other person is saying. Therefore during this exercise you are not allowed to say the word, 'I.'"
3. Announce, "Each of you has three clothespins, and at the end the person with the most clothespins wins a gift. To collect a pin from another person, you must hear him or her use the word, 'I,' and you must be the first one to claim a clothespin from that person. If you hear someone say, 'I,' whether it is the person you are in direct conversation with or a person nearby, you have the opportunity to collect only one clothespin from that person."
4. Invite learners to stand and find a partner. They may change partners as often as they wish.
5. When 5 to 10 minutes has elapsed, announce that the activity is over and invite learners to sit down in their chairs.
6. Identify the person with the most clothespins. If it is a tie, randomly select from the winners. Ask that person to select a gift from the ones you have provided.

Educator secrets

Join in the activity with the learners to hone your skills and to be an inclusive class member.

64

7. Collect the clothespins for reuse.
8. Distribute the Take the Communication Challenge questions sheets, and ask the learners to answer the questions.
9. Foster a discussion on the importance of listening, focusing on others, and the challenge of being an effective communicator.

65

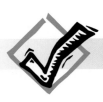

Take the Communication Challenge
QUESTIONNAIRE

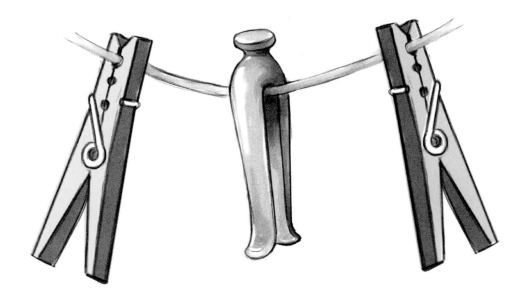

DIRECTIONS: Read the following questions, and answer them based on the clothespin activity that was just completed. After this, feel free to converse with the instructor about your experience.

1. Who had the most pins in the room?
2. How do you account for your own success in collecting clothespins?
3. What scenes stand out in your mind during this activity?
4. At what point were you pulled into the exercise?
5. What events or experiences do you associate with this activity?
6. What came through to you as being important?
7. What did you learn about yourself during this activity?
8. What did you learn about others?
9. If you had to give this activity a title, what would you name it?
10. To what degree was it difficult or easy for you to really listen to the other persons talking?
11. What accounted for it being easy or difficult?

Are You Listening?

Sandra Stokes, RN

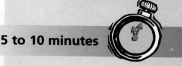

5 to 10 minutes

Preparation

1. Copy the Are You Listening? Question Sheet (one for each participant).

Implementation

1. Divide your class into pairs.
2. Ask one person to be person "A" and the other to be person "1."
3. Give the pairs a moment to decide who is "A" and who is "1."
4. Person "A" will have 60 seconds to tell person "1" what they are most proud of in his or her life. Person "1" is to be the best listener in history. He or she cannot interrupt, but can smile, nod, or show interest nonverbally.
5. Start the timer for 1 minute. When time is up, announce that Person "1" must now become the worst listener in history. Announce person "A" should continue to talk.
6. Now it is time to switch roles. Person "A" becomes an excellent listener for 60 seconds; then at the instructor's cue, he or she becomes the worst listener. Person "1" becomes the talker.
7. Debrief the session with the questions on the Are You Listening? Question Sheet.

Tool box
- **Are You Listening? Question Sheet for each learner**
- **Clock or stopwatch that measures 1 minute**

Educator secrets
Notice the volume in the room will increase during the minutes when participants are demonstrating poor listening skills. People sometimes feel they must talk louder to be heard.

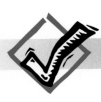

Are You Listening?
QUESTION SHEET

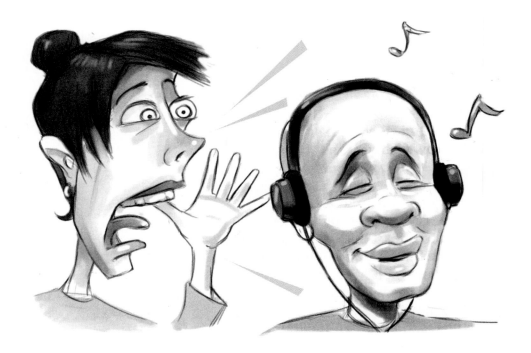

DIRECTIONS: Read the following questions, and answer them based on the listening activity that was just completed. After this, feel free to converse with the instructor about your experience.

1. What did it feel like to be really heard and listened to?
2. What was it like to talk and know the other person was not attentive?
3. What was an example of the worst listening behavior you observed?
4. What was an example of the best listening behavior you observed?
5. How does this compare to real-life situations? Do you ever find yourself preoccupied?
6. What are some of the ways to become a better listener?

Dress Me Up!

Cheryl Burnette, MEd, RN

Preparation

1. Spread out your collection of dress up items on a table so that everyone can see the items.
2. Load the camera. If using a Polaroid camera, lay the pictures on a table to fully develop so that everyone can see them. If using a digital camera, hook it to a laptop to rotate through the pictures during classroom breaks.

Implementation

1. Ask the participants to count off by fours to form a team of four people. It is nice to mix the groups so that participants have a chance to meet new people.
2. Each four-member team will have an opportunity to work together to dress each other up. Select one team to start.
3. Encourage them to pose each team member for his or her own individual picture.
4. The rest of the team must encourage their members by cheering them on and offering support.
5. Only one team at a time is to dress up, but the rest of the large group is instructed to watch, enjoy, and think of what items they may want to use when it is their turn.
6. When the team is ready, the facilitator takes a picture of each team member.

Continued

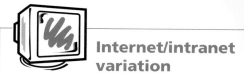

Internet/intranet variation

Post pictures on Intranet or e-mail them back to the learners a month after the program to remind them of their day.

Tool box
- **Dress-up items:** can include anything (but some things that seem to go over well include feather boas, masks, beads, Halloween stuff, scarves, crowns, plastic sunglasses, plastic fangs, and old children's costumes or toys).
  Note: The sillier the items you select, the more fun it is for all.
- **Polaroid or digital camera**
- **Film for the Polaroid camera, if applicable**

Educator secrets
High-energy music playing in the background can increase energy during this activity. Have fun!

Dress Me Up!—cont'd

7. After each team has dressed up and had their pictures taken, the group decides on what will be done with the pictures. If the class participants are from many departments, each person can keep his or her own picture.

8. If the group is all from one department or area, recommend using all the pictures with their permission on a poster board to keep in the lounge as a reminder of their day together.

9. Debrief this activity by discussing trusting your team, being willing to expose yourself to being in a vulnerable position, and how nice it is to have team support.

Preceptor and Peer Coaching Bingo

Vivian Jefferson, RN, MSN

Length of lecture on this topic, approximately 15 to 30 minutes

Preparation

1. Copy the Preceptor/Peer Coaching Bingo Sheet, one per participant.
2. Ready your lecture notes.

Tool box
- **Preceptor/Peer Coaching Bingo Sheet**
- **Lecture notes on preceptor/peer coaching**
- **Small prizes**

Implementation

1. Distribute the Preceptor/Peer Coaching Bingo Sheet to each participant along with a pen or pencil.
2. Invite the learners to listen to your lecture about roles and responsibilities and to circle the words on the page as they hear them.
3. Bingo is achieved when all the words are circled, as in blackout bingo format.
4. Take all the completed Bingo cards and place them in a random drawing.
5. Award a prize to the winner of the random drawing.

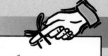

Educator secrets
You can make a variety of cards with words in different places for fun and excitement.

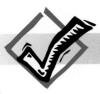

Preceptor/Peer Coaching Bingo Sheet

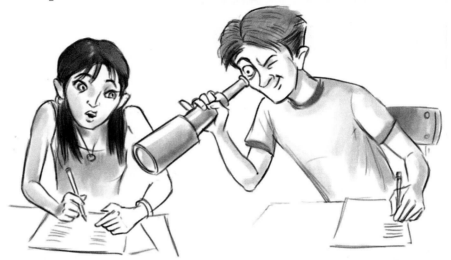

Roles	Coach	Change	Resolution
Coping	Orientation	Job	Mission
Values	Feedback	Socialize	Results
Fear	Belonging	Resistance	Competency
Peer	Department	Loss	Challenge

TOPIC: Communication, collaboration, negotiation, teamwork, building trust

Blindfolded Bath Salts

Cheryl Burnette, MEd, RN

30 to 45 minutes, depending on the size of the group

Preparation

1. Place all the ingredients, mixing containers, bath salt containers, gloves, essential oils, and food coloring on a separate table from the team's table.
2. Leave all the ingredients in their original containers for transport and the activity. Do not divide the ingredients!

Tool box

- One plastic rectangular container—able to hold approximately 2 gallons—per each small team (for mixing bath salts)
- Ingredients for bath salts can vary, but generally for each four-member team should include the following:
  - Two large boxes of baking soda
  - One box of kosher salt
  - One bag or box of Epsom salts
- Essential oils: Several types, including a relaxing type of scent and an invigorating scent. (Essential oils are readily available on-line and may be available at health stores in your area.)
  - Lavender and tea tree oil (These oils are for relaxing and healing. Use no more than 10 to 15 drops combined. Using more than this will just make it stronger smelling.)
  - Peppermint and either orange or lemon (These oils have a stimulating type of scent. Again, use no more than 10 to 15 drops for the mix.)
- Gloves to mix the bath salts
- One blindfold for each group of four to five participants
- One set of food coloring (so learners will be forced to share)
- One container for the bath salts per each small team (such as 1-quart zip lock bags or inexpensive plastic containers)
- A table for supplies

Note: Thousands of recipes exist for bath salts, but using these ingredients work best. You can't mess them up; if they are not in exact amounts, it is fine.

Educator secrets
This may sound complicated but really is not. Participants enjoy the fun of this activity and have a gift to take home when it is over.

Continued

Blindfolded Bath Salts—cont'd

Implementation

1. Invite the group to count off by fours. (This activity works best in teams of four to five people.)
2. Distribute one mixing container for each team.
3. After the group is formed, have them pick a spot at a table for their work area.
4. Tell them that in this activity they will make bath salts that they can take home.
5. Ask the groups to each choose someone on their team who will be blindfolded, and explain that is the only person that can actually touch the ingredients and make the salts.
6. They may at any time switch the blindfold to another team member; but again, only the blindfolded person may touch the ingredients or talk to anyone outside of their small group.
7. Distribute a blindfold to each group.
8. Display the bath salt ingredients, the essential oils, gloves, and food coloring on a special table (separate from the group table).
9. Purposely have less of the bath salt ingredients than you need for each group, so they will have to collaborate and negotiate.
10. Instruct them to make the bath salts by writing down how much they will need for each group.
11. Each group can decide if they want to use food coloring to color their bath salts, essential oils, or both. If they choose either of them, suggest they use gloves.
12. If they use food coloring, recommend they use 10 to 15 drops.
13. If they choose to use essential oils, recommend they use no more than 10 to 15 drops in their mixing container.
14. The teams have to collaborate and negotiate using the oils and colors, because you have purposely provided only one set of each.
15. The team will have to lead the blindfolded person to the table to collect the ingredients and to the other tables to borrow items if needed (because only the blindfolded person does the collaborating and negotiating). He or she is also the only one who touches any of the things used to mix the bath salts.
16. Circulate around the groups to answer any questions that arise.
17. When a group has finished and may be sitting idle, ask them if they can do something else or help another group. This encourages them to think about assisting others and sharing resources.
18. After all groups are finished, debrief the participants about the skills just used (i.e., communication, collaboration, negotiation, teamwork, trust building).

Last to Stand N'Awlins Style

Iris Trahan, RN, BSN, CCRN

Preparation

1. Write questions about the content you want to review. Include multiple-answer and single-answer questions.
2. Set up the table or cart in the front of the room with the raffia table skirt attached.
3. Place the bells on the table or cart.

Implementation

1. Divide your group into two teams with equal numbers on either side of the classroom setup. Ask them to think of a team name and write it on the signs you distribute to them.
2. Individuals of each team write their names on small index cards you provide.
3. Collect the index name cards in the wicker basket assigned to their group. Place the basket on the cart or table in front, with the team name sign in front of it.
4. Give each team 5 minutes to choose their "Big Kahoona," who will become the leader. This person dons the Hawaiian-style shirt.
5. The Kahoonas come up to the table. The course coordinator selects one of the prewritten questions that requires only one answer. (You could describe a patient scenario, asking for the probable patient diagnosis based on the signs and symptoms given.)
6. The first Kahoona to ring in with the correct answer wins the "N'Awlins necklace" for his team. The other team now has to get rid of one of its members.
7. A name is pulled from the wicker basket of the losing team. The course coordinator then calls out the person's name and states, "The group has spoken." He or she then escorts the person off by carrying the tiki light from the table.

Tool box
- Tropical theme items for party or thrift stores
- Two extra-large tropical-print (i.e., Hawaiian) shirts
- Raffia table skirt and tropical trees
- Table or cart
- N'Awlins style Mardi Gras necklace
- Two wicker baskets
- Index cards
- Two tabletop tropical tiki lights
- Shell necklaces
- Gummy worms
- Signs with team names
- Two desk bells from an office supply store

Continued

Last to Stand N'Awlins Style—cont'd

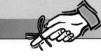

Educator secrets

You might replace the shirts with bandannas in case Big Kahoonas are unwilling or unable to fit into their shirts. This avoids embarrassment for any team player.

8. If the Kahoona who rings in first answers the question incorrectly, the other team wins and the losing team has to get rid of one of its members by drawing names.

9. To continue the game, the losing team has to answer a question requiring multiple answers. Each team member in a row takes a turn giving a different answer. If the team is unable to give all the correct answers, the remaining number of answers is the number of team members who are selected to leave. (Example: Name 6 signs and symptoms of congestive heart failure. If the group members are only able to answer four, two team members are out.)

10. The game continues until the time limit is reached. The winning team is the group with the most standing members left.

11. Option 1: The winning group gets a prize (e.g., shell necklaces, tropical pencils). The losing team gets to pass around the gummy worms and eat bugs.

12. Option 2: The coordinator states everyone in health care is the last standing, and everyone gets a small prize.

Saying Good-Bye

Sandra Stokes, RN

1 hour for a group of 10 people (If more people are present, estimate about 6 minutes per person.)

Preparation

1. The employee who is leaving meets with his or her supervisor. He or she is asked to identify simple, individual "gifts" appropriate to give each of the remaining employees and to bring those gifts on a specified date to a closing event. The gift could be something simple but meaningful, such as a box of tissues (because the two employees shared a certain time when they each needed a lot of tissues). Alternatively, it might be a pair of scissors, because the remaining employee was forever losing his pair. It could be a green leaf from a tree symbolizing how the remaining employee helped the one leaving to grow.

2. The supervisor contacts all the remaining team members to ask that they select individual meaningful gifts to be shared with the employee who is leaving. One employee may give a bag of marbles with the explanation, "You have worked so hard here. Take time to play in your new job." Another may be a stamped envelope with the verbal explanation that, "You have been my best friend here, and I want to hear from you as soon as you are settled in your new job."

3. Because of the nature of the sharing, it is important to have this activity in a quiet and private space.

4. Play reflective music as participants enter the room.

Tool box
- One small, meaningful memento from each learner for the person leaving
- One small, meaningful memento from the person leaving for each of the remaining team members
- Quiet and private space for the event
- Reflective music and player

Implementation

1. Once participants have gathered, the supervisor asks, "Will one of you begin the exercise by sharing your first memory of the employee who is leaving and anything you want the person to know.

2. Each person shares as he or she presents the simple gift and explains its symbolism. It is important (both as a collective team and as individuals), to have a structured method to remember how the leaving employee joined the team, to share meaningful stories of the relationship orally, and to perhaps heal old wounds in the process.

Continued

Saying Good-Bye—cont'd

3. After the employees share, the leaving employee presents his or her gifts to the individual team members with the explanation of the symbolism in the gift presented.
4. Employees are asked to stand and form a circle with the leaving employee in the middle. If appropriate, employees join hands in the circle. The honored employee is told, "The circle symbolizes our team and how important you have been to us. We grieve that you're leaving us. Please remain in the circle as long as you need to, and when you are ready, break through the circle and take several steps toward the exit. Doing so symbolizes that we will not be the same team without you. Thank you for the time you have spent with us and the contributions you have made to this team."
5. When the employee is ready, he or she steps out of the circle and moves to the door. Often strong emotions surface during the entire process, and there needs to be a short time for employees to recover. This activity can be done 2 to 7 days before the person leaves.

Variation

1. A facilitator rather than a supervisor can conduct this activity.
2. Delete physical gifts and use only verbal remembrances.
3. Record with prior permission and give a copy to everyone at the end.

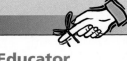

Educator secrets
This exercise can bring healthy closure to all involved. It can encourage private sharing of what the relationship has meant to the one leaving and the ones staying.

Internet/intranet variation
People who work as teams on the Internet can all meet in a chat area to share remembrances. Instead of physical gifts, meaningful wishes may be offered and posted on a bulletin board if desired.

Did You "Drop the Ball?"

Susan Bosold, MS, MA, RN

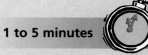

1 to 5 minutes

Preparation

1. Obtain hackey sack.
2. Set the timer to 1 minute.
3. Select candy or other small prizes.
4. Personalize the debriefing questions and copy or print them.

Implementation

1. Explain that the goal of the activity is to see how many catches the participants can complete without "dropping the ball."
2. At the word, "Go," the instructor tosses the ball into the audience, who then toss it to each other.
3. Each time someone catches it, the audience counts consecutively, "One, two, three, four, five...." until either the ball is dropped or 60 seconds is up, whichever comes first.
4. Post the "record" tosses to date.
5. Each time the audience improves, each member either gets a Smartee (roll of candy) or 3 minutes added to their next break or small gift.
6. Use the Debriefing Questions on the ready-to-use sheet to stress important learning points.

Tool box
• Hackey sack ball
• Timer (60 seconds)
• Smartees roll candy (optional) or small prizes
• Did you "Drop the Ball?" Debriefing Questions

Variation

1. The previous "tosser" may not catch the ball. For instance, if Ann throws the ball to Andy, Andy may not throw it back to Ann. If Ann does catch it, the game continues but the catch is not counted.
2. With a larger group of students, specify that each student may only catch the ball one time, until all students have caught the ball. In that way, they also have to remember who has already had the ball. They can coach each other (which should be encouraged). The game continues if a student catches the ball more than once, but "duplicates" cannot be counted. The goal is to complete more tosses than in the previous round.

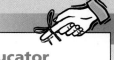

Educator secrets
Notice the sense of calm or urgency and watch the fun.

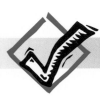

Did You "Drop the Ball?"
DEBRIEFING QUESTIONS

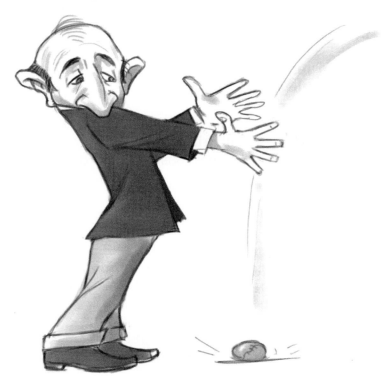

1. During the activity, to what did you pay attention?
2. What did you think would enhance your score?
3. What did you notice compromised your efforts?
4. Do those considerations apply to other team activities and, if so, how?
5. How does this compare to situations that occur on your job?
6. How does this compare to situations that occur in your life?

Command Keepers

Michele L. Deck, RN, MEd, BSN, LCCE, FACCE

Use throughout your regular class time; the activity adds only the time for the explanation and involvement, approximately 5 to 10 minutes

Preparation

1. Review your notes before class and decide which "commands" to assign to learners. These should be ones that are usually repeated several times by the instructor.
2. Ready the index cards and bag by setting them up in the front for your later use.

Implementation

1. Explain to the group that as they learn to use the computer or the equipment you are demonstrating, each person will have one step they are responsible for remembering and explaining to others.
2. Begin your class. For example, when instructing a class on computer use, you could say, "The first step in using the computer is to log in. Sue, you will be the person who has to remember the log in command. First we click here, then scroll there, then press enter." Then you could say, "Barry, please be in charge of the patient charting function. The way we do this is to scroll down to the unit name, press enter, and click on the correct patient record. Look, the computer is asking for us to log in again. Sue how do we do that?" Sue then takes the group through the log in process.
3. Each person is assigned a function to remember and repeat after the initial explanation by the instructor. Every time that function happens, the person then cues the rest of the class.
4. Once everyone is confident of his or her command, you can introduce command scramble.
5. Invite each learner to write down the name of his or her command on an index card. Collect the cards in the paper bag and mix them up.
6. Ask the participants to pick a new command from the bag. This is the one they are responsible for until class is over.
7. If teaching pumps or other equipment, each person is responsible for one part of the setup and use, such as the "thread the pump" procedure and the "how to reset alarm" functions.

Tool box
- Index cards
- Paper bag

Educator secrets
This activity encourages ownership and interest in a class that might only have been presented in uninterrupted lecture format.

3 minutes to explain; carried out in usual class time allotment

Cup of Understanding

Michele L. Deck, RN, MEd, BSN, LCCE, FACCE

Preparation

1. Prepare the sets of cups before class.
2. Place the cup stacks at each person's place before class begins, or hand them out to learners at the door.

Tool box
- **One set of paper or plastic cups (in red, green, and yellow) per learner**

Implementation

1. Explain to the learners that they have each received three cups, stacked one atop the other.
2. As long as they understand the instructor's presentation, they are to leave the green cup atop the stack. This is the learner showing, "I understand everything and am on board with the information presented so far."
3. If they need immediate help (stat!) they are to place the red cup atop the stack. This is the learner showing, "Stop what you are doing and come here immediately." (This is great during computer classes or equipment class when they mess up a preset series or travel in cyberspace to areas that are private.)
4. If they just have a general question, they are to place the yellow cup atop the stack. This is the learner showing, "When you have a chance, I have a question for you."
5. Begin your class content. Periodically check the color of the cups and respond appropriately.

Educator secrets
Reuse and recycle the cups from one class to another. This idea also prevents confusion in learners.

Variation

1. Distribute one set of cups per small team of three to five people. Select a leader who is responsible for keeping the cups visible and changing them as need arises in the group.
2. It is possible for teams to teach each other when one person is confused. This decreases the amount of time the instructor spends in clarifying. If no one understands, the cups are used as signals.

Popcorn Buckets

Michele L. Deck, RN, MEd, BSN, LCCE, FACCE

5 to 15 minutes

Preparation

1. Precount the bags and index cards into sets to match the number of participants you will have on each team.
2. Place markers with the bags and index cards, so that team members can share them.

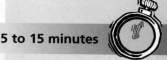

Tool box
- **One brown paper bag for each participant and instructor**
- **One index card per person**
- **Thick markers**

Implementation

1. Divide your class into small teams of three to six members.
2. Recruit a volunteer from each small team to come up to the front to get needed supplies you have precounted.
3. Ask each person to use a marker to place his or her own name on his or her paper bag.
4. Ask everyone to open the bag and stand it in front of his or her place.
5. You do the same to model it.
6. Ask each person to obtain an index card. Instruct the group to fold the index card in half, pressing on the fold.
7. Ask the group to fold it in half repeatedly, for a total of three folds, while you demonstrate.
8. Request that everyone open the card and reveal the eight segments on the index card delineated by folds.
9. Have the participants tear on the folds to create eight small pieces of paper.
10. Explain that the papers will be the makings of "popcorn" that will go into everyone's bucket.

Internet/intranet variation

You can invite participants to send positive comments to others in a course at a specified time interval, such as evaluation time.

Educator secrets

A written note of encouragement can be reread and enjoyed for a long period of time. Many people keep these and reread them on hard days at work.

Continued

Popcorn Buckets—cont'd

11. Invite the learners to write one nice, positive comment to each person on their small team. They are to then crumple it and drop it in that person's bag.

12. Everyone will have extra pieces of paper left. Invite them to write comments for as many others in the class as they like and to sneak it into those bags at breaks.

13. State that no one is allowed to read the comments in their bags until the class is over and they are off the grounds of your facility.

14. Be sure to display your bucket and to place "popcorn" in as many bags as you can.

15. This makes a wonderful closing event at the end of orientation or graduation. You can collect the bags and send them back to attendees 3 to 6 months after class has ended. Many of them will need it more at that time than at the end of class.

Variation

1. A nurse I met suggested this to her staff for a patient's family whom they had grown close to over a long illness. Each staff member wrote a memory, a nice comment, or both about the deceased, and the bag was presented to the family as a keepsake.

The Weakest Think

Michele L. Deck, RN, MEd, BSN, LCCE, FACCE

Preparation

1. Copy The Weakest Think ready-to-use page (one per small group or learner).
2. Personalize the scenarios to your facility or situation.
3. Cut the options into strips of paper. You will have eleven strips of small print and the three strips of headings.
4. Place each set (one page cut out) into an envelope.

Tool box
• **One copy of The Weakest Think ready-to-use page per small group or learner**

Implementation

1. Distribute one envelope set to each person.
2. Challenge learners to place each of the various scenarios under one of the following categories: *All the time, It depends,* or *Never in a million years.*
3. Allow three to 5 minutes for everyone to finish.
4. Discuss under which heading each scenario was placed and why.
5. Clarify guidelines to facility rules or patient management situations.

Variation

1. Put people into small groups and provide one set of strips for each group. They must then discuss the options and come to a group consensus.
2. Observe if team members are just going along with a dominant person, or if they think the idea is not sound and didn't say so.

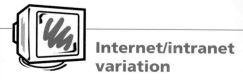

Internet/intranet variation

Place in on-line bulletin board area to foster discussions

Educator secrets
Many of the people who go to nursing school have been in jobs in which a poor decision would not result in a life-threatening situation. For example, electrical safety is paramount when a patient's life-saving equipment is hooked to an extension cord, but it is not when a small appliance (e.g., a blender) is hooked to an extension cord.

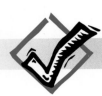

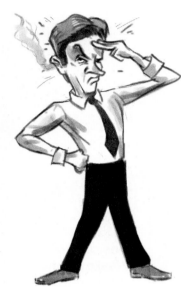

The Weakest Think

All the time

It depends

Never in a million years

You go to your supervisor to report a safety hazard. He or she ignores you. Two weeks later, do you report it to someone higher up?

You see a small piece of trash on the floor. Do you pick it up?

You accidentally stick yourself with a needle after drawing blood, but after you have emptied the syringe and flushed the line with saline. Do you report it?

Your computer monitor is on a desk that is too low. Do you use it anyway?

The machinery you are working with begins to make an odd noise. Do you keep using it?

You are at home and need an extension cord for holiday lights. You find one that doesn't have a grounding plug. Do you hook the three-prong device to the two-prong plug?

Your coworker is not following procedure but has found a faster way of doing a job. Do you tell your supervisor?

You are dispensing medications. You drop a pill on the floor that cost $35 each. Do you pick it up and give it to the patient?

Your supervisor asks you to sign a report as a witness to an accident. You were too far away to have seen the details. Do you sign it?

You haven't been officially trained to use a new piece of equipment. It is very similar to one you have used in the past. Do you fill in for the trained person?

Have you ever skipped wearing your personal protective devices?

Ask It Basket

Michele L. Deck, RN, MEd, BSN, LCCE, FACCE

This takes the place of question-and-answer time

Preparation

1. Label the bag or a basket.
2. Place it on a table that is centered along the right or left side of the room.
3. Place stacks of index cards at each learner's place.

Tool box
- Basket or bag labeled, "Ask It Basket" on a side table
- Index card

Implementation

1. Explain that you would like to invite questions at any point during your class.
2. Ask the learners to simply write each question on an index card and pass them all to the person closest to the basket. He or she will then place the cards in the "Ask it basket."
3. At intervals or when you need a change of pace, go to the basket and select a question or two to answer.
4. The questions are all anonymous, so learners feel free to ask more questions than if they had to ask them in front of the group.
5. If you do not know the answer to a question, leave it in the basket and get the answer at a break or lunch. Say something like, "Three questions are in the basket. Let me answer two now, and I'll save the other for later."
6. If someone asks a question scheduled later in your lecture, place it back in the basket to answer it at an appropriate time so that you don't get off track.
7. After class has ended, you might publish a list of the questions and answers and send them back to the group by e-mail as a review of important content.

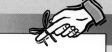

Educator secrets
This allows you to keep track of questions in a written format. Often when instructors are asked questions out of sequence with the course material, they say they will answer the question later. They sometimes forget to get back to it until class has ended.

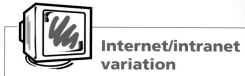

Internet/intranet variation

Invite people to post questions as they have them when going through Internet course. Compile most frequently asked questions for later use.

Which Hat Are You Wearing?

5 to 7 minutes

Michele L. Deck, RN, MEd, BSN, LCCE, FACCE

Tool box

- **One set of visors (in red, green, and blue) per learner**
- **Clock or stopwatch**

Preparation

1. Use this idea when 90% to 100% of the audience is not happy about attending your class and is vocal about it when arriving (possibly mandated groups).
2. Place a set of three visors or hats (in red, green, and blue) at each participant's table area as they arrive.
3. Ready your own set of visors.
4. Set the clock or stopwatch for 2 minutes.

Implementation

1. Explain that each person has received a special set of hats that serve a specific purpose.
2. Invite each learner to put on his or her red hat. Place yours on your head as well.
3. Display the clock set for 2 minutes.
4. Tell the group they have 2 minutes to discuss, "Isn't it awful that…" They are to converse with those around them until the alarm sounds.
5. Once the alarm has sounded, invite each learner to place the green visor on his or her head. Reset the clock for 2 minutes. Place your green hat on as well.
6. Tell the group they have 2 minutes to discuss, "Isn't it great that…" They are to discuss only the positive aspects of life until the alarm sounds.
7. Once the alarm has sounded, invite them to wear the blue hats from now on. These are known as the "learning hats," and it is time for everyone to learn. Place your blue hat on your head as well.
8. Later, if a topic comes up that stirs negative feelings, you can repeat the red, then green sequence, but for 30-second time intervals instead of 2 minutes. End with everyone returning to the blue hats.
9. It is critical that the negative ventilation happen first, followed by the positive words. If you reverse this, you will not get the same positive results.

Educator secrets

Substitute less expensive items for the hats, such as construction paper, name tags, ribbons, scarves, rubber bands, nonlatex balloons, and markers.

Seven Reasons We Should Not Have Come to Class Today

Michele L. Deck, RN, MEd, BSN, LCCE, FACCE

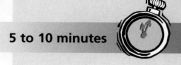

5 to 10 minutes

Preparation

1. Use this idea when 90% to 100% of the audience is not happy about attending your class and is vocal about it when arriving (possibly mandated groups).
2. Tear off sheets from the flipchart pads and place them in a convenient place for learners to take when directed.
3. Place markers with paper.

Implementation

1. Place learners into teams of three to six members.
2. Select a leader in a fun, random way (example: The person who is the tallest).
3. Invite the leader to get one sheet of paper and a marker or two from your displayed supplies.
4. Set the timer for 2 minutes.
5. Challenge the small groups to compete against the other teams in the room to create a list of seven reasons they should not have come to this class today in only 2 minutes or less (on the front side of the paper only).
6. Begin by saying, "Get ready, get set, go!"
7. Call time at 2 minutes. Poll the group to see how many teams were able to list seven reasons.

Tool box
- **Blank flipchart paper**
- **Markers**
- **Tape or adhesive to hang chart pages on the wall**
- **Clock or stopwatch**
- **Small prizes**

Educator secrets
Set the stage for the small groups to compete against each other. The natural competition will cause them to think up positive reasons so they can beat their peers.

Internet/intranet variation

Have groups compete to post a list of negatives and positives in a bulletin area. Invite individuals to vote for the best list (the one they feel deserves to win course points or small prizes).

Continued

Seven Reasons We Should Not Have Come to Class Today—cont'd

8. Tell the group you have prizes you will award after part two of the activity. They are to turn the paper over to the backside of the paper and label it, "Seven Reasons Why We Should Have Come to Class Today."
9. Any group that can list seven positive reasons they should have come will receive prizes.
10. Begin by saying, "Get ready, get set, go!"
11. Call time at 2 minutes. Poll the group to see how many teams were able to list seven reasons.
12. Distribute prizes as team leaders hang the chart pages with the positive sides (reasons to come) showing to the class for the rest of the day.

A Penny for Your Thoughts

Michele L. Deck, RN, MEd, BSN, LCCE, FACCE

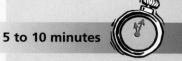

Preparation

1. Bring a coin or two with you to class.

Implementation

1. Break your learners into small teams of three to six people per team.
2. Ask each person to reach into a pocket, purse, organizer, or briefcase and find one coin, any denomination will do. They can borrow a coin from those around them if desired.
3. Select a leader of each small group. The leader might be the person with the highest number of coins with them.
4. Get your coin ready.
5. Instruct the participants to turn their coin to the side with the profile visible. This is the side with the minting year engraved on it. They must read the year on the coin to themselves.
6. Each person must then think of something that happened to him or her in or around the year on his or her coin.
7. Tell your coin memory first to model it.
8. Invite team leaders to facilitate a sharing of the individual's memories from the years depicted on their coins with their small team.
9. Remind the participants to put away their money or return it to original owners at the end of the activity.

Tool box
- **One coin for each learner. (Ask them to bring their own coins.)**
- **One or two coins for the instructor.**

Internet/intranet variation

At the beginning of an Internet course, invite learners to post in a bulletin board area their coin memory, whether personal memories or professional developments. This way people are no longer anonymous screen names.

Educator secrets
This activity helps people to feel comfortable with new acquaintances by offering opportunities to network.

Continued

A Penny for Your Thoughts—cont'd

Variation

1. Ask the participants to discuss how nursing practice has changed since the year on their coins. (Example: In 1979 we allowed new dads only 1 hour to hold their newborns in the evening from 8 to 9 PM. No other visitors were allowed in the baby's presence. Now with multiple visitors, mothers and newborns have rooming in!)
2. Have the group identify a significant occurrence that happened in the year by selecting a team coin. (Example: In 2003 the new HIPAA guidelines changed our unit by....)

Vehicle Memories

Michele L. Deck, RN, MEd, BSN, LCCE, FACCE

3 to 10 minutes

Preparation

1. Precount supplies and distribute them before class begins.
2. Draw your vehicle so that you can model this activity when explaining it.

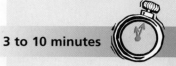

Tool box
- **One piece of paper per learner**
- **One marker per learner**

Implementation

1. Break your learners into small teams of three to six people per team.
2. Select a group leader in a fun way, such as the person who came the farthest distance to class today.
3. Ask your participants to think back to the very first motorized vehicle they ever drove.
4. Using the markers, they are to draw a simple sketch of the vehicle.
5. Show your picture and tell your vehicle memory.
6. Invite the group leaders to facilitate a sharing of stories and pictures in the small team setting. Give them a time limit of 2 to 5 minutes, depending on the number of participants in a group.

Educator secrets
In this activity, everyone is the same for a few minutes. It doesn't matter whether you are the CEO or a member of the housekeeping department; everyone has the same sort of feelings about first driving experiences.

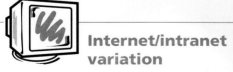

Internet/intranet variation

At the beginning of an Internet course, invite learners to post their vehicle memories in a bulletin board area. This way people are no longer simply anonymous screen names.

Give Each Other a Hand

Michele L. Deck, RN, MEd, BSN, LCCE, FACCE

5 to 10 minutes

Preparation

1. Test the paper by writing on it with the marker before learners come to class. It is essential that the markers do not bleed through.
2. Distribute one sheet of paper and envelope per participant, and include yourself.
3. Place masking tape on the back of the chairs or desk (one piece per person).
4. Set up the music so it is ready to play.

Implementation

1. Each person is to trace his or her hand on the sheet of paper with a marker. Model this yourself.
2. Ask learners to help each other to tape this piece of paper on their backs. Ask someone to attach yours.
3. When the music begins, they are to travel through the room, giving each other a hand. This means everyone will write one nice, positive statement or comment on as many "hands" as they can in a 3-minute period.
4. Start the music. Write on as many hands as you can in the period.
5. At 3 minutes (or more if you'd like), turn off the music and ask everyone to take their seats.
6. Invite participants to self-address the envelopes you provided.
7. Ask the participants to pair up and take the "hands" off each other's backs, fold them, and place them in the envelopes of the people to whom they belong. They are to seal the envelopes.
8. Collect the envelopes.
9. Distribute the envelopes back to the learners after class has ended (i.e., 1, 3, or 6 months after).

Tool box
- One sheet of high-grade copy paper (8$\frac{1}{2}$ × 11) per learner
- One sheet for the instructor
- Mr. Sketch brand water based markers
- Masking tape
- Upbeat music and music player
- One envelope per learner

Educator secrets

Participants are initially surprised they will not get to read the comments in class. However, they look forward to receiving these after class has ended—a time when they are likely to need some positive reinforcement and feedback.

Internet/intranet variation

Ask learners to write a nice comment for each person in your on-line class and e-mail it to you. Collate the comments and e-mail each person their list of comments after the course is over.

Graduate Each Other

Michele L. Deck, RN, MEd, BSN, LCCE, FACCE

3 to 5 minutes

Preparation

1. Distribute a certificate or diploma face down on each learner's place. Make sure no one has his or her own. Instead, be sure that each learner has someone else's certificate or diploma.
2. Set up the music.

Implementation

1. Explain that when the music begins, they are to stand and find the person whose certificate they have received. They are to shake that person's hand, pat them on the back, and congratulate them for completing the course. They are to personally, "graduate" them by presenting them with the written proof.
2. Someone will then find him or her and also perform the graduation ceremony.
3. Once they have presented and received a certificate, they are to sit back down at their place.
4. Turn on the music.
5. Once everyone is back in his or her seats, turn off the music.
6. Congratulate everyone.
7. Dismiss your class.

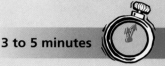

Tool box
- **One certificate of attendance or diploma per learner**
- **Appropriate music, such as "Pomp and Circumstance"**
- **Music player**

Educator secrets
This is a joyful and unusual way to distribute paperwork that is learner focused. A great sense of anticipation exists as people wait to see who has their certificate, and everyone gets equal attention.

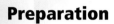

2 to 4 minutes

Flag This!

Michele L. Deck, RN, MEd, BSN, LCCE, FACCE

Preparation

1. Scan your written materials, and divide the content into these categories:
   a. Need to know—Must master and remember by the end of class without help
   b. Need to find—Must be able to find this information in a certain situation or know who to ask
   c. Nice to know—Interesting information, but not critical to the first two previously mentioned categories (Sometimes this is the history or the technology behind the content.)
2. Place the three colors of tape flags at each person's place.

Educator secrets

This prevents over-load when learners see a large volume of written informa-tion. They are given clear expectations of what can be done in a short time frame with a large volume of information.

Implementation

1. Explain that the materials for the course are extensive and will not all be covered in class.
2. Ask each learner to select red tape flags and to place them on the pages, sections, or both you are announcing. When you are fin-ished the need to know content flagging, ask the learners to find the yellow flags.
3. Announce they are to "let their fingers do the walking through the yellow pages" and put yellow tape flags on the pages, sections, or both you are announcing. Just like the yellow pages of a phone book, they can look things up in this section. When you are fin-ished the need to find content flagging, ask the learners to find the blue flags.
4. Read the list of blue flag pages, sections, or both. Tell your group these are the nice to know sections. These are interesting, and they are invited to read them on their own time outside of class. Class time will not be spent in these sections.

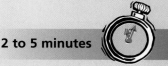

TOPIC: Review and reinforcement of information, teamwork, energy builder

Book Ball

Michele L. Deck, RN, MEd, BSN, LCCE, FACCE

2 to 5 minutes

Preparation

1. Select a time in your class when energy is low.
2. Place scratch paper in an easy-to-reach location for class members.

Implementation

1. Ask your learners to stand and form small teams of three to six members.
2. Have one person from each team crumple the scratch paper into a tight ball.
3. Invite the learners to pick up their "paddle," which is their hand-out, book, or notebook from the class.
4. Explain that when you say to begin they are to hit the crumpled ball back and forth to team members. The object of the activity is to keep the ball in play.
5. If someone misses, he or she must tell the member of the small team one thing he or she has learned so far in class. After hearing the person's statement, play begins again.
6. At the end of about 2 minutes, ask everyone to sit back down to resume the session.

Variation

1. Set the goal that each team must spell out a word without miss-ing. If your class is about infection control, they have to each spell a letter in "infection" while hitting the ball. For example, the first person hits and says, "I," the next hits and says, "N," and so on.
2. If someone misses, he or she must tell the member of the small team one thing he or she has learned so far in class. After hear-ing the person's statement, play begins again.
3. Play continues until each small group has reached their goal and then sits down.
4. It is interesting to watch groups problem solve in this situation.

Educator secrets
This activity reener-gizes a tired group and will usually generate some laughter, fun, and playfulness.

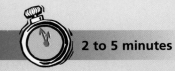

2 to 5 minutes

Count Off

Michele L. Deck, RN, MEd, BSN, LCCE, FACCE

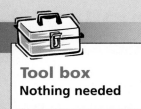

Tool box
Nothing needed

Preparation

1. Decide where you will insert this activity in your class.

Implementation

1. Announce to your class that you will be conducting a one to 20 count off in the room. In a minute the instructor will begin by saying, "One." Someone else in the class continues by saying, " Two." Then someone else says, "Three." The same person cannot say two numbers in sequence. If two or more people try to speak at once, the sequence must start over.
2. Give them no time to think and immediately say, "One."
3. When two or more people are speaking the numbers simultaneously, stop them and start over with "One."
4. Repeat this process two or three times.
5. Announce to the group you will now leave the room for 30 seconds, and when you return, you will begin the process again in hopes of success.
6. Leave the room. A leader will emerge from the group and formulate a plan.
7. Return to the room and begin by saying, "One."
8. Most groups will be able to complete the set of 20 this time. If necessary, you can go out again and return 30 seconds later.
9. Facilitate a discussion of why it is important to plan, problem solve when faced with a challenge, and work together as a team. Compare this to challenges they each face on the job every day.

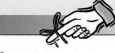

Educator secrets
No two groups ever solve this challenge the same way. Watch what leadership styles are exhibited and who listens or argues.

TOPIC: Nonverbal communication, team building, energy builder

Line Up By...

Michele L. Deck, RN, MEd, BSN, LCCE, FACCE

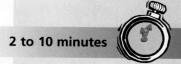

2 to 10 minutes

Preparation

1. Select the criteria you will use to ask the class to form lines.
2. Clear an area of the room to make some space for teams to move.

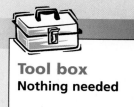

Tool box
Nothing needed

Implementation

1. Ask your learners to stand and form small teams of six to eight members.
2. Invite them to find some space in the room where they can form a line easily, without obstacles.
3. On your signal they are to line up in order, based on the criteria you give them at the time. They are to do this quickly in an effort to beat the other teams in the room.
4. Announce they are to line up by height. The first team that finishes is polled and they each state their height verbally.
5. Encourage everyone to beat this team in your next round.
6. Announce they must line up by day and month of their birth (NO YEARS), but cannot talk while lining up.
7. There will be some confusion and excitement as they figure out another communication system other than talking. Poll the team that finishes first for the day and month of their birth. Ask what system they used to communicate.
8. Announce they must line up by the number of siblings they have, but they can't use their hands in any way.
9. There will be more confusion and excitement as they figure out a way to communicate other than talking and using their hands. Poll the team that finishes first for the number of siblings. Ask what system they used to communicate.
10. Ask the groups to sit down. Briefly discuss the difficulties of non-verbal communication and working together toward a goal without verbal communication.
11. Other categories might include the following: how many miles away from the class they live, how many years they have been in their current job, or the number of pets they own.

Educator secrets
This can get to be fun and energy producing. Enhance the feeling of competition between the teams so that they are hurried in forming lines.

99

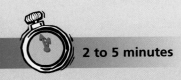

2 to 5 minutes

Strike a Pose

Michele L. Deck, RN, MEd, BSN, LCCE, FACCE

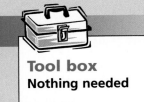

Tool box
Nothing needed

Preparation

1. Prepare your discussion points on nonverbal communication and the difficulties involved with it.

Implementation

1. Invite your group to stand and quickly get into pairs. If an uneven number of participants is present, ask the person without a partner to be the room observer. (He or she must travel around the room watching people, reactions, comments, and so on to report back to the large group.)
2. Ask the pairs to stand back to back but not to touch.
3. Explain that on the count of three, they are to turn around to face their partners, to strike a pose, and to hold it. You will offer further instructions then.
4. Say, "One, two, three, strike a pose!"
5. Declare that anyone who just happens to match the pose of his or her partner should sit down. Those who did not match should turn back to back again with their partners.
6. Say, "One, two, three, strike a pose!"
7. Declare that anyone matches the pose of his or her partner may be seated. Those who did not match should turn back to back again with their partners for the last time.
8. Say, "One, two, three, strike a pose!"
9. Invite everyone to be seated.
10. If there was a room observer, elicit feedback as to what he or she observed.
11. Ask for a show of hands of those that matched the first time each person posed. Emphasize that they did not even know the goal was to match, but they did. This represents the people in our lives with whom we find it easy and natural to communicate. Our styles match, so much understanding exists and little confusion occurs.

Educator secrets
You will notice laughter and energy generated by this activity. Keep it moving fast between rounds.

12. Ask for a show of hands of those who changed their pose the second or third time to try to match their partner's previous pose. This represents how we sometimes change our communication style or delivery to try to communicate more effectively with those who are different from us. Sometimes it works and sometimes it does not.

13. Ask for a show of hands of those that did not match in three tries. This represents how even though we both might be trying, it is difficult to communicate with everyone effectively. Sometimes a difference in style exists; sometimes it is a difference of timing. Nonverbal communication is just as important and confounding as verbal communication.

Aerobic Quiz

Michele L. Deck, RN, MEd, BSN, LCCE, FACCE

2 to 5 minutes

Tool box
- **One chair for each learner, including the instructor**
- **Yes-or-no or true-or-false questions from your content**

Educator secrets
At the end of this activity, people are awake, alert, and ready to learn more information and skills. It also allows you to see if someone is consistently answering incorrectly so that you can clarify certain points with the learner. Move through the questions quickly, balancing between true and false answers.

Preparation

1. Make sure you, the instructor, have a chair to sit in for this activity.

Implementation

1. Explain that each person will simultaneously experience an "Aerobic Quiz."
2. Ask each person to stand and to place the back of his or her chair against any wall in the room. You model the same behavior in a spot where you can be seen and heard.
3. Ask each person to stand in front of his or her chair, facing away from the wall, with the back of his or her legs touching the front of the chair.
4. Explain you will ask a series of questions. If the answer for them is yes or true, they are to briefly touch their rears to the chair and then stand erect again (demonstrate as you explain this move). If the answer is no or false, they are to just remain standing.
5. Caution that if it gets too aerobic for anyone in class, they can sit down and just raise a hand for yes or true.
6. Begin with a sample question, such as, "Is your heart beating?" You will go up and down and so should the entire class.
7. Continue with some fun questions first such as:
   a. Do you have a pet?
   b. Do you like pizza?
   c. Have you ever been on a cruise?
   d. Have you ever owned red shoes?
   e. Do you like to travel?
8. Shift the questions to content questions such as:
   a. True or false. The best way to wash your hands is to use only water.
   b. True or false. A paper fire calls for the use of a CO_2 extinguisher.

The Wave

Michele L. Deck, RN, MEd, BSN, LCCE, FACCE

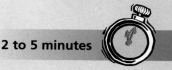

2 to 5 minutes

Preparation

1. Decide the order in which the wave will travel through your class.
2. Obtain a chair for yourself if you do not have one.

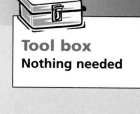

Tool box
Nothing needed

Implementation

1. Ask how many of the participants have ever seen or experienced the wave at a sporting event. Explain each person will be experiencing the wave in this class.
2. Request that everyone push their chairs back a bit from the table, so they will not hit their knees when it is their turn to stand.
3. Position your chair in front of the room.
4. Map out for participants (verbally or with a picture) who will start the wave and how it will move through the group—one person at a time standing, raising his or her arms, and then sitting back down. I like to start the wave in the back corner, so it ends with the instructor in the front.
5. The designated person in the back begins the wave. It travels through the room and ends with the instructor. Encourage the group to applaud their efforts.
6. Now, challenge the group to experience the "Learning Wave."
7. Each person thinks of something he or she has learned in class that can be expressed in one, two, or three words total. Give everyone about 15 seconds to look through their notes or think of something.
8. Instruct them that when the learning wave begins, not only do they stand and raise their arms as before but also they are to say what they have learned at the same time.
9. The designated person in the back begins the wave. It travels through the room and ends with the instructor. Encourage the group to applaud their efforts.
10. If you want to raise the level of difficulty, set a rule that no one can repeat what anyone has already said.

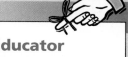

Educator secrets
This is a fun review of content and reenergizer of sleepy people.

Continued

The Wave—cont'd

Variation

1. Divide your group into teams. Have the teams perform the wave and speak in unison the content learned.

Mixing Experience Shows

Michele L. Deck, RN, MEd, BSN, LCCE, FACCE

5 to 10 minutes

Preparation

1. Place one long strip of masking tape across the front of your classroom.
2. Identify the person at the session with the most experience and the least experience on your topic. If you get a roster ahead of time, you can look it up. If people "just show up" for your class, meet each one at the door and ask them how much experience he or she has on your topic. Again, your goal is to identify just the two extremes.

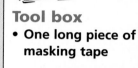

Tool box
- **One long piece of masking tape**

Implementation

1. Introduce the class to the person with the most experience. For example, "When Jerry came in today, I found out this is the twenty-fourth year he has worked as a nurse in our facility and the twenty-fourth year he has taken this CPR recertification class. I am going to ask Jerry to stand on this end of the tape, so he represents 24 years of experience."
2. Introduce the class to the person with the least experience. For example, "When Sue came in this morning, I found out she is a new graduate, this is her first job as a nurse, she has been here 2 weeks, and this is her first CPR recertification class. I am going to ask Sue to stand on the opposite end of the tape representing 1 year of experience with CPR."
3. Ask the rest of the class to line up as to where their experience level puts them on the tapeline. Let them compare their experience levels as they come to and stand on the line.

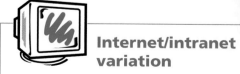

Internet/intranet variation

Divide your class in teams by experience, and have them coach each other during team projects.

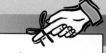

Educator secrets
This helps learners of varying experiences to feel valued and not bored or overwhelmed.

Continued

Mixing Experience Shows—cont'd

4. Stand in the middle facing the people on the line.
5. Ask the two people from either end (Jerry and Sue) to come to you in the middle of the line and pick two people from the center of the line. These four people are a work team and must now sit together.
6. Ask the two people from left at either end to step to you in the middle of the line and pick two people from the center of the line. These four people are a work team and must now sit together.
7. Continue assigning work teams in this manner.
8. Each team now has the wide variety of experience. At intervals, encourage them to coach each other and work as a team to get everyone's knowledge and skills up to standard.
9. The people who have the most experience can act as mentors and coaches to the newer people. Their experience is valued and they know it.
10. The less experienced people don't feel as overwhelmed or intimidated, because they have peers they can count on.
11. The people from the middle of the line have the role of mediator and act as "voices of reason" if a dispute occurs.

Step In

Michele L. Deck, RN, MEd, BSN, LCCE, FACCE

5 to 10 minutes

Preparation

1. Distribute one or two small pieces of scratch paper to each learner.
2. Ask each person to write a yes-or-no question he or she would like to have everyone in the room answer. This might be a topic they want to network on, or something about which they are curious. State that everyone will answer the questions, including the person writing it. Give some examples if they look puzzled.
3. Collect the papers in the paper bag and mix them up.

Implementation

1. Ask the group to form a circle in the back or front of the room. Join in the circle yourself holding the bag.
2. Explain that when you read a question, if the answer is true for someone, he or she is to take one step into the circle, pause, and then step back out.
3. Read the first question. (Example: "Do you know a good resource on pain management?" or "Have you ever been to Europe?")
4. Continue until all the questions from the bag are asked.
5. Encourage people to network with those whom they identified during break times.
6. Clap for everyone and ask all participants to resume sitting.
7. Continue with your class.

Tool box
- **One paper bag**
- **One or two small scratch sheets of paper per participant**

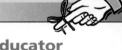

Educator secrets
It is sometimes a good idea to preview the questions before you begin.

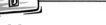

3 to 5 minutes

Who Do You Look Like?

Michele L. Deck, RN, MEd, BSN, LCCE, FACCE

Preparation

1. Decide your answer to the questions you will pose to them, so you can model the activity.
2. Create an overhead or screen with the Who Do You Look Like? ready-to-use page.

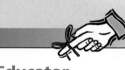

Tool box
• **Who Do You Look Like? ready-to-use page**

Implementation

1. Divide your group into small teams of three to six people.
2. Select a leader in a fun way, such as the person having the shortest hair.
3. Display the questions, and ask everyone to mentally answer them.
4. Begin by telling who people say you look like.
5. Explain that if you could look like anyone in the world, who it would be.
6. Tell the group if you could be anyone other than yourself for 24 hours, who it would be and why.
7. Direct the leader to make sure all members answer the three questions aloud to share with the small team within a 4-minute period.

Educator secrets
How you model and enjoy this one sets the tone for the group.

Internet/intranet variation

Ask learners to post their responses on a bulletin board area of the course, so they are no longer anonymous screen names.

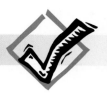

Who Do You Look Like?

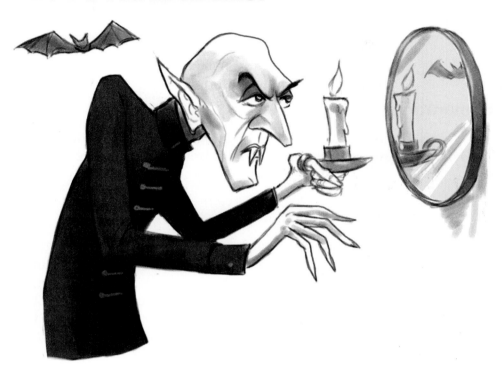

1. Who do people sometimes say you look like?
2. If you could pick anyone in the world, who do you wish you looked like and why?
3. If you could be anyone for 24 hours only, who would it be and why?

TOPIC: Review and reinforcement of information, teamwork, closing activity to orientation or graduation

10 to 30 minutes, depending on how many participants you have

Receiving Line Review

Michele L. Deck, RN, MEd, BSN, LCCE, FACCE

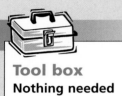

Tool box
Nothing needed

Preparation

1. Use this idea when a class is ending as a way to say goodbye, review important information, and to bring closure to the group.

Implementation

1. Begin by asking everyone in your class to reflect on everything they have learned and to pick out the single most important thing they will use when on the job.
2. Think of one thing you the instructor learned from this class.
3. Stand in the front of the room. Encourage the person sitting in the last row to come up and share his or her idea with you.
4. Shake hands with the person as he or she approaches. Tell him or her what the one thing you have learned and will use is. Ask what his or her idea to use is. Thank the person for coming to your class. Ask the person to stand to your left.
5. Invite the next person in the last row to come to the front.
6. Shake hands with the person as he or she approaches. Tell him or her what the one thing you have learned and will use is. Ask what his or her idea to use is. Ask the person to do the same with the person to your left. They shake hands and share ideas.
7. The person then moves to the left of the person to your left.
8. Continue with this process until everyone has joined the line. This forms a "receiving line" of sorts and invites participants to say their own goodbyes to each member of the class while you are orchestrating a sneaky review of important content that is participant driven.
9. When the last person passes those in the beginning of the line, they are free to leave class when they are ready. This holds true for everyone in the line.

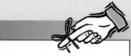

Educator secrets
This allows the instructor to hear what the learners felt was the most valuable information gained in class. It also allows you to tell each of them good-bye.

Confetti Cards

Michele L. Deck, RN, MEd, BSN, LCCE, FACCE

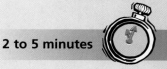

2 to 5 minutes

Preparation

1. Place the index cards where each group easily obtains them.

Tool box
- One index card per group or person

Implementation

1. Divide your class into small teams of three to six people.
2. Select a leader of the group in a fun way. For example, the leader is the person who got up earliest this morning.
3. Explain the topic of your class. For example, "Today's class is all about infection control. What is one question or challenge your group has about this topic that you would like answered or solved?"
4. Ask the group leader to write the question or the challenge that the team decides upon on the index card.
5. Instruct the group that when the challenge or question is addressed or answered, they are to tear up the card (or make confetti out of it) and then celebrate by clapping and cheering, no matter what is happening in class at that moment.
6. When you see a celebration going on, stop and ask the group what was their question and how was it just answered. This is an opportunity for a participant-centered review.
7. During class and breaks, travel around the room reading the confetti cards, and then gear your teaching toward answering them.
8. At the end of the class factor in 3 to 5 minutes to answer any intact and unanswered confetti cards.

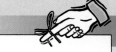

Educator secrets
Use some of the same words on the cards in your lecture. For example, if the card says, "What are the most common causes of infection in the nursery?" you would begin your sentence with, "The most common causes of infection in the nursery this year are...."

Continued

Confetti Cards—cont'd

Variation

1. If you have small groups, ask each person to write a question or challenge, and use these to see when participants are understanding and absorbing important information.

Internet/intranet variation

Ask learners to post questions on a bulletin board before they begin, and then answer them for all to see in this area when they have discovered the information in the course. This creates a great section for most frequently asked questions.

Race List

Michele L. Deck, RN, MEd, BSN, LCCE, FACCE

3 to 5 minutes at end of class

Preparation

1. Distribute one sheet of flipchart paper and two markers to each small team.
2. Set the timer to 3 minutes.

Tool box
- Flipchart paper
- Markers
- Small prizes
- Timer or stopwatch

Implementation

1. Divide your group into small teams of three to six people.
2. Select a leader of the group in a fun way. For example, the leader is the person who is wearing the largest watch.
3. Have the leader recruit two people to write on the paper and position it so that they can easily reach it.
4. Explain to the group when time begins they will have 3 minutes to create the longest list in the room of everything they have learned in class today. Stress that quantity is important, because you know they will all be quality answers.
5. Announce the teams can use their notes, but only two people can be writing on the paper.
6. Say, "Ready, Set, Go!"
7. At the end of the 3 minutes call out, "Stop."
8. Ask the writers to count up the number of items on their team's list.
9. Award prizes or points based on number of entries written. Teams with the most points choose first, but all receive a small prize.

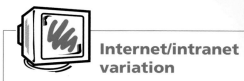

Internet/intranet variation

If you are conducting synchronous chats, small teams can submit their lists when completed.

Educator secrets
This allows you to see if the learning points you stressed were seen as important to learners. It also serves as a content review before class ends.

2 to 5 minutes

Question Quest

Michele L. Deck, RN, MEd, BSN, LCCE, FACCE

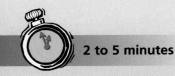

Tool box
- Stopwatch or timing device

Preparation

1. Set the clock to 3 minutes.

Implementation

1. Divide your group into small teams of three to six people.
2. Select a leader of the group in a fun way. For example, the leader is the person who is wearing the most rings.
3. Tell the groups they have 3 minutes to look through all of their notes from class to discover any unanswered questions they might have before class ends.
4. Instruct the team to answer any of the questions that come up in the small group if they can. If they cannot, the leader is to record the question, and it will come before the entire room at the end of the period. (This way the learners can answer the easy questions themselves.)
5. Ask the leaders to share questions that were unanswered by their teams.
6. Answer the questions generated but that remain unanswered.

Educator secrets
This allows for better quality questions to come to the attention of the whole class. Instead of having questions like, "What was the third fill-in-the-blank question on page seven?" The questions are more complex and compelling.

Internet/intranet variation
In synchronous chats, have people work together in small discussion groups to do the previously mentioned activity.

114

Stretch Yourself!

Michele L. Deck, RN, MEd, BSN, LCCE, FACCE

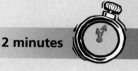

2 minutes

Preparation

1. Just to be sure, write on a piece of sample flipchart paper to test that the markers you are using do not bleed through to the back of the paper.
2. Hang a clean piece of paper high on a flat wall using the tape or adhesive (the flipchart pads that have the port it material are perfect for this activity).

Tool box
- **One sheet of flipchart paper**
- **Two different colored Mr. Sketch Markers that do not bleed through paper**
- **Tape or adhesive to hang paper on wall**
- **Step stool to hang paper high on wall**

Implementation

1. Recruit two volunteers for this activity. Ideally, there should be a height difference between them.
2. Ask each to select a different colored marker.
3. Escort both participants to the chart paper hanging high on the wall.
4. Quickly say, "Staying on the paper, please draw a line across it as high as you can."
5. Each person draws a line.
6. Instruct with these words, "Now, again staying on the paper I want you to REALLY draw a line as high as you can!"
7. Some participants will stand on their toes, others will grab a chair and stand on it, others will jump while drawing, etc.
8. Point out to the group the visual differences in the two sets of lines.
9. Stress to the group that this class will ask them to "stretch themselves and their abilities."
10. Thank the volunteers and begin your class content.

Educator secrets
The second line can be drawn in several ways. You can make analogies to these throughout your class; for example, "Sometimes it is smart to find a tool that will help us reach our goals, such as the way Mary used the chair."

115

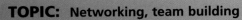

Crossing Life Lines

Michele L. Deck, RN, MEd, BSN, LCCE, FACCE

5 to 10 minutes

Preparation

1. Draw your five-event life line in preparation for class to begin.
2. Keep your pictures very simple.

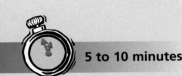

Tool box
- **One piece of paper per learner**
- **One pen or pencil per learner**
- **Flipchart paper or overhead projector film for the instructor**

Implementation

1. Divide your group into small teams of three to six people.
2. Select a leader of the group in a fun way. For example, the leader is the person who has the most letters in his or her last name.
3. Explain to the group that each person will have an opportunity to share five events from his or her life with his or her teammates. The person is free to choose which events. One can start at birth or any point on the line. Each person picks five—no more and no less.
4. Model the activity by displaying and explaining your life line.
5. Ask the group leaders to facilitate this activity in their small teams. Tell everyone the group has 7 minutes to complete the activity as a team.
6. Watch your leaders and make sure most if not all teams finish this activity before moving into other content areas.
7. Encourage the participants to network with the people they have met and found some commonality with the life lines.

Educator secrets
Draw stick figures and simple pictures to model this activity. (See example on next page.)

Internet/intranet variation
Ask learners to complete this activity on home page areas for participants to network.

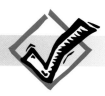

Crossing Life Lines
LIFE LINE EXAMPLE

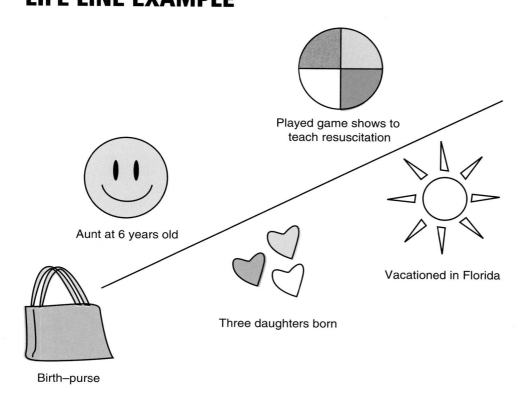

Played game shows to teach resuscitation

Aunt at 6 years old

Vacationed in Florida

Three daughters born

Birth–purse

Verbal Explanation

You may notice I have drawn my life on the upswing, because I like to believe that every day gets better and better to be alive.

Purse

I was born in New Orleans at Mardi Gras time. I am the fifth child of my parents, who were driving to the hospital when they were caught in parade traffic. My father dropped my mother off at the emergency room door and went to park the car. They placed my mother on a stretcher; she put her purse down by her knee, and I was there too. By the time my father parked the car, I was already in the nursery.

Face

I was 6 years old when my nephew Mike was born, and all my friends were impressed that I was already an aunt.

Continued

Crossing Life Lines—cont'd

Hearts

This represents the birth of my three wonderful daughters, who have taught me to be a mom.

Wheel

This represents over 17 years ago, when I began to teach using games to show how to resuscitate others. No one was doing that back then.

Sun

My most recent vacation was to Orlando, Florida.

The Best Teacher I Ever Had

Michele L. Deck, RN, MEd, BSN, LCCE, FACCE

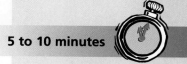

5 to 10 minutes

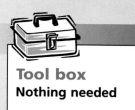

Tool box
Nothing needed

Preparation

1. Think about which story you will share with the group. I like to choose someone the group can relate to; for example, if teaching a group of nurses, I will share a story about someone who taught me much about being a nurse. If teaching teachers, I share a story about my eighth grade teacher, etc.

Implementation

1. Divide your group into small teams of three to six people.
2. Select a leader of the group in a fun way. For example, the leader is the person whose birthday (day and month, NOT YEAR) is closest to the current date.
3. Tell your story to the group. Stress what made them a great teacher and the importance of what he or she taught you that holds true today.
4. Ask the leader to facilitate this activity for the group. He or she is responsible for everyone having a turn in the short time frame you allow (e.g., 3 to 4 minutes).
5. If desired, you can ask one or two participants to share their best teacher story with the entire class. Make sure to stress what made them effective.
6. Begin your content with everyone alert, awake, in a positive frame of mind, and ready to learn.

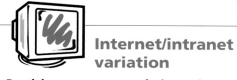

Internet/intranet variation

Participants can post their stories on a bulletin board area to facilitate networking.

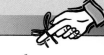

Educator secrets
Be sincere in relating what made your teacher the best you ever had.

Continued

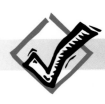

The Best Teacher I Ever Had
EXAMPLE STORY

I remember Ms. Carbo was the 3 PM to 11 PM charge nurse of the labor and delivery unit where I worked as a new graduate nurse. From my memory she was a career nurse. To my young mind this meant that she was old fashioned and I was a shiny new graduate. The first shift I worked with Ms. Carbo, she made me check all the expiration dates on the drug supplies throughout our large unit. I remember thinking it was busy work when she made me do that same task when I came on every evening for months. After the first month, I told her I had made a chart of all the expiration dates and no longer needed to check them. She disagreed, so I continued checking for 3 months. She also taught me how to mop a delivery room, clean and flash instruments, and set up sterile supplies for a delivery room—all chores in my mind that were the responsibility of the housekeeping crew and our technicians. At the time I thought it was not necessary, because I was a NURSE!

I wasn't working 6 months when I suddenly had a decisive moment concerning her reasons for being so hard on me. A patient came in with an imminent emergency, and we were busy. There was not a clean delivery room or setup ready for a Cesarean delivery, which was what this patient and her baby needed immediately. We all pitched in and had the Cesarean delivery going within 7 minutes. The baby was fine, but the mom was having some serious problems. When the anesthesiologist turned to me and asked for epinephrine (a drug rarely used on any delivery unit), guess who was the only person in the room who knew where it was? It was I, of course, because I had checked it for the expiration date for 3 months.

I have a wonderful appreciation of the job Ms. Carbo did in teaching me to be a competent and confident nurse. She was teaching me every job there was to do on the unit, so I was never afraid or unaware of what to do when emergencies did happen. She was an excellent teacher, and I want to thank her for making me the nurse I am today.

PART 4

Instant Tools for Curriculum and Continuing Education

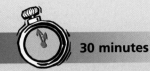

30 minutes

Take a Bite!

Rhonda Scott-Foertsch, RN, BSN

Tool box
- **Large brown paper bag with pictures of feed on it**
- **Note cards (5 × 7 inches)**
- **Answer key**
- **Tape**

Preparation

1. Make note cards with the digestive organ or structure's name on one side. On the other side, list the functions of that organ or structure.
2. Number the cards in the same order that the digestive organs or structures affect a bite of food.
3. Prepare the answer key to match the note cards.

Implementation

1. Explain to the class that they will be guessing which digestive organ or structure is being described by its function or functions.
2. Number the cards in the order that the digestive organs or structures affect a bite of food.
3. Have each participant draw a card out of the bag. Keep drawing until all the cards are given out.
4. Call for the cardholder of card No. 1 to come to the front of the room. Ask him or her to read the functions on the back of the card.
5. Challenge the class to say which organ or structure is being described.
6. Tape the card to the board and call for card No. 2. Continue in order until all cards are posted in the correct sequence.

Educator secrets
Review and reinforce content in a fun, interactive way.

Pressure Ulcer Prevention

Gino Chisari, RN, MSN

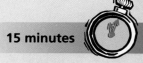

Preparation

1. Prepare a talk on pressure ulcer formation.
2. Deliver a talk on the causes of pressure ulcer formation, and stress immobility factors.

Tool box
• Clock in view of presenter or stopwatch

Implementation

1. During your talk on pressure ulcer formation, invite participants to volunteer to sit on their nondominant hand for 15 minutes to simulate some of the effects of immobility.
2. Time the sitting period to no more than 15 minutes, and announce when it is over.
3. After the 15 minutes have each participant inspect his or her hand for color, sensation, and mobility changes.
4. Hold discussion on these changes while relating immobility factors to pressure ulcer formation.

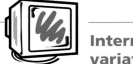

Internet/intranet variation

In an on-line course, users could sit on their nondominant hand while completing this information in module form on a computer.

Educator secrets
Participants should be given a choice of whether or not to comply.

Pass the M&Ms

20 to 30 minutes   Gina M. Ankner, MSN, RN, CS

Tool box

- Enough plain chocolate M&M candies for each participant to take at least three.
- A container and scoop that allows a few M&Ms to be retrieved from it with minimum contact with participants' hands.
- One blank piece of paper and pen or pencil per participant
- Overhead with the definitions of "close-ended," "open-ended," "leading," and "biased" questions
- Overhead with the definition of "subjective" and "objective" data
- Overhead projector
- 12 8^1/$_2$ × 11-inch signs, each with one of the months of the year written on it

Preparation

1. Place the M&Ms in the container with a scoop.
2. Prepare the overhead transparencies of definitions.
3. Prepare the 12 signs (indicating the months of the year) to hang on the walls about 4 to 5 feet apart.

Implementation

1. Distribute a piece of paper and a pen or pencil to each participant.
2. Pass around the container of M&Ms, and instruct each participant to take as many as they wish, with a minimum of three per person.
3. Once each participant has M&Ms, instruct him or her to write down one question per M&M. The questions can ask anything and should be directed toward someone they have just met.
4. Invite the participants to break into groups according to their birth month and stand by the sign on display for their month.
5. Once in groups, instruct participants to introduce themselves to someone they do not know and ask this person their questions, listening carefully to the answers. The partner does the same.
6. Ask the participants to return to their seats.
7. Ask the group if anyone would like to read their questions. Did anyone ask a funny question? A question they didn't expect? A thought-provoking question? A question they wouldn't answer? What types of responses did they get—short and to the point or long stories? Did a question lead to discussion of a related topic?
8. Reveal the overhead of the definitions of "close-ended," "open-ended," "leading," and "biased" questions. After a brief discussion of the definitions, ask each participant to label his or her questions as "close-ended," "open-ended," "leading," and "biased." Ask for an example of each from the group.

9. Display the overhead of the definitions of "subjective" and "objective" data. After a brief discussion of the definitions, ask each participant to recall the answers they received and label his or her questions as likely to elicit "subjective" or "objective" data. Ask for an example of each from the group.

10. Conclude with an explanation of times during a client assessment when each type of question is appropriate, when it is not, and when and how a health care provider can collect subjective data and objective data.

Volume Ventures

5 to 10 minutes

Erin Davis, MS, MEd, RRT

Tool box
- **Medium-sized balloons**

Preparation

1. Lecture on lung volumes and capacities, or ask the learners to read about the subject.

Implementation

1. Have the learners blow up balloons with a small volume if air in the balloon. Explain this represents residual volume in the lungs.
2. Next, have a learner blow in and out of the balloon, not letting the original volume out of the balloon. Explain this represents tidal volume.
3. Finally, invite learners to blow into the balloons to full capacity. Explain this represents total lung capacity.

Educator secrets

Don't let the learners empty all the air out of the balloons. Be careful no one hyperventilates.

What's My Disease?

Mary LaBiche, MEd, RRT
Erin Davis, MS, MEd, RRT

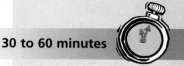

30 to 60 minutes

Preparation

1. Select several diseases that learners have studied or researched.
2. The learners need to know the definition of the disease, as well as symptoms, treatment, x-ray findings, diagnosis, and other pertinent information.
3. Create an index card with the name of a disease, patient age, diagnosis, and where the patient is presenting (e.g., emergency department (ER), hospital).

Tool box
- **Reference material**
- **Index cards indicating a fictitious patient's name, age, and diagnosis**

Implementation

1. Learners are given an index card with the name of a disease, patient age, diagnosis, and where the patient is presenting (e.g., ER, hospital).
2. Recruit a volunteer to stand in front of the class with his or her card indicating the diagnosis of the patient.
3. Ask the student to play the role of a patient with that diagnosis. They are allowed only to answer questions other students ask. No additional information should be given.
4. The questioning students need to ask the patient's chief complaint, age, symptoms, and chest x-ray findings and interview the patient until they can determine a diagnosis. The following is an example in which patient will refer to the learner who has been assigned to act as someone with a disease process and student will refer to the learner who is interviewing the patient and asking questions.

Note: The patient is given a 3- × 5-inch card saying, "You are a 65-year-old patient with a history of COPD [chronic obstructive pulmonary disease] who presents to the ER with SOB [shortness of breath] and pneumonia."

Educator secrets
It is important to have the instructor present to make sure the answers are correct and to guide the learners. Instructors may need to encourage students to use interviewing skills more adeptly. This activity can also be used to teach interviewing skills, analytic thinking, and knowledge of disease processes.

Continued

What's My Disease?—cont'd

Student: How old are you, and are you "male" or "female?"
Patient: I am a 65-year-old male patient.
Student: Where are you at this time?
Patient: I am in the ER.
Student: What brings you to the ER? What is your chief complaint?
Patient: Shortness of breath.
Student: What are your vital signs?
Patient: RR [respiration rate] 35 bpm, HR [heart rate] 120, BP [blood pressure] 150/95.
Student: Do you have a fever?
Patient: Yes, 102°.
Student: What are your breath sounds?
Patient: Decreased with crackles on the left lower lobe.
Student: Are you cyanotic?
Patient: Yes.
Student: What is your SaO_2?
Patient: 85%.
Student: Do you have a history of smoking?
Patient: Yes.
Student: How much did you smoke?
Patient: Two packs a day for 25 years.
Student: What is your medical history?
Patient: I have a history of lung problems and shortness of breath.
Student: How long have you had these problems?
Patient: About 10 years.
Student: What are your symptoms?
Patient: What do you mean?
Student: Do you cough and how often?
Patient: I cough almost every day.
Student: Do you produce any sputum, and can you describe it?
Patient: Yes, and now it is yellow and thick.
Student: Have you been diagnosed with chronic bronchitis?
Patient: Yes, I have, but now it's worse.
Student: Tell me how it is worse.
Patient: I have a pain in my left side, and it is harder to breathe.
Student: What are your x-ray results?
Patient: The left lower lobe is consolidated; the rest of the x-ray is consistent with COPD.
Student: Do you have pneumonia on your lower left lobe?
Patient: Yes.

Simulating the Work of Breathing

Mary LaBiche, MEd, RRT
Erin Davis, MS, MEd, RRT

10 minutes

Preparation

1. Instruct the learners on the work of breathing through an artificial airway or airway obstruction (as in asthma).
2. This activity will easily demonstrate the increased work of breathing.

Tool box
- Straw
- Nose (optional) clips

Implementation

1. Have the learners breathe through a straw for 30 seconds to 1 minute with nose occluded (use a nose clip or have the participants hold their nose).

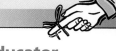

Educator secrets
Make sure the only air learners breathe is in through the straw.

15 to 20 minutes

What I Meant Was...

Gina M. Ankner, MSN, RN, CS

Tool box
- **One piece of blank paper and a pen or pencil per participant**
- **Two jars of peanut butter**
- **Two jars of jelly**
- **Two loaves of bread**
- **Two plates**
- **Two knives**
- **Two spoons**
- **Some napkins**
- **Desk or tabletop**

Educator secrets
The more literally you take the instructor's written steps, the more dramatic the point will be made that one should not assume anything. To save money, you can use one jar of peanut butter, one jar of jelly, and one loaf of bread. Have the two teams share.

Preparation

1. Keep the peanut butter, jelly, bread, plates, knives, spoons, and napkins hidden from view.
2. Clear off a tabletop large enough to accommodate the food and paper goods listed previously.

Implementation

1. Distribute a blank piece of paper to each person, and ask him or her to write out directions for making a peanut butter and jelly sandwich.
2. When everyone has finished, call up four volunteers to the front of the room. They should bring their directions with them.
3. Divide the four participants into two teams of two. Ask one to volunteer to be the instructor and the other to be the chef.
4. Reveal the supplies, and place them on the desk or tabletop.
5. Ask the first team's instructor to read the first step in their directions exactly as written, and explain that the chef must do exactly what the instructor has read. For example, if the instructor reads, "Put the bread on the plate," the chef must take the whole loaf of bread and place it on the plate, because the instructor did not say to open the bread bag, take out two slices, and then place them on the plate.
6. Have the second team do the same, with the instructor reading exactly from their directions.
7. Continue to go from the first team to the second team, with each team completing one step at a time. In some cases one team may not get further than their first or second step.
8. When each team has completed their sandwich as much as possible, ask the participants how this relates to documentation.

130

9. Explain that often the instructor (or person documenting a client's plan of care) knows exactly what interventions he or she would like implemented for the client; however, he or she does not convey that clearly in the documentation. Instead, the documenter assumes that the chef (another health care provider) will know what was intended and will "fill in the blanks" if necessary. For example, if the chef did not open the loaf of bread, the instructor may have commented, "What I meant was..." or "Well of course the chef would do that first." When one assumes the comprehension level and the actions of another, he or she risks improper implementation secondary to miscommunication of the intended plan of care.

10. Remind participants to reread their documentation after it is written to ensure that what they have intended to convey in writing is clear to the reader, whether they are documenting future care needed or care they have provided.

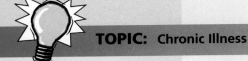

TOPIC: Chronic Illness

Chronic Illness Crossword Puzzle

Sandy Wilbanks, RN, BSN, CDE

10 to 15 minutes

Preparation

1. Make a copy of the ready-to-use Chronic Illness Crossword Puzzle for each participant.
2. Use this as an introduction to the lesson or review after the lesson.
3. Make sure all participants have a pen or pencil.
4. Make a copy of the answer key.

Tool box
- **Chronic Illness Crossword Puzzle**
- **Pens or pencils**
- **Answer key**

Implementation

1. Distribute the large or small crossword puzzle.
2. Challenge your learners to complete the puzzle as individuals or as teams.
3. If energy and attention are low during your lesson presentation, stop and let your participants engage in this energizing activity.
4. Crossword puzzles can act as pre- or posttests, and they can also be sent out days or weeks after the lesson as reinforcement of important concepts.

Variation

1. Use a poster printer copy machine to turn the crossword into a poster-sized image.
2. Plan for groups of two to six to discuss and fill in a poster-sized copy of the crossword puzzle before or after your lesson.

Educator secrets
If you have different ability levels in your session, pair learners to maximize benefits to all participants.

Internet/intranet variation
Include this crossword puzzle on-line in a course as a pretest or posttest.

132

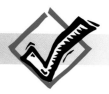

Chronic Illness Crossword Puzzle

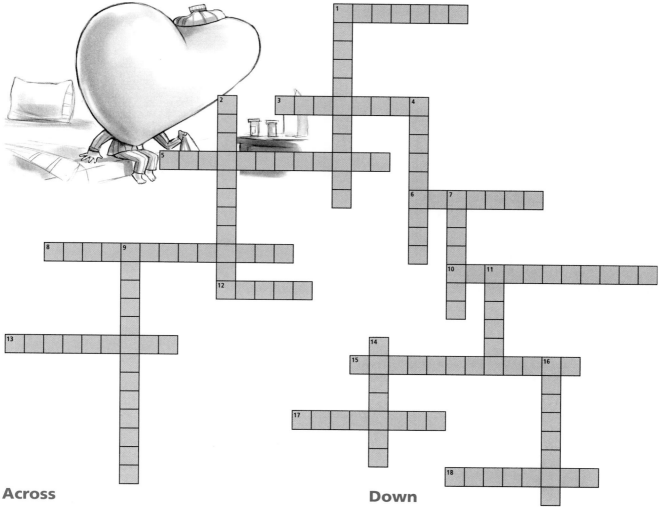

Across

1. A condition that affects daily functioning for more than 3 months per year
3. The leading cause of blindness in the United States
5. BP higher than 140/90
6. Body mass index (BMI) greater than 26
8. Often felt by patients with a chronic illness
10. Poor lifestyle choices, or genetic predispositions *(two words)*
12. A chronic illness lasts for _____
13. Most chronically ill individuals live and work in their _____
15. The goal of health care for its chronically ill members
17. A feeling often associated with self-induced diseases
18 A reduction in functional status

Down

1. Having more than one chronic illness
2. A feeling associated with being chronically ill
4. A grouping of diseases that includes diabetes, hypertension, obesity, hyper-lipidemia, and heart disease *(two words)*
7. Not the largest group affected by chronic illness
9. An important social factor influencing patient outcomes
11. A label placed by society
14. What chronically ill individuals feel they lose
16. Measurable results

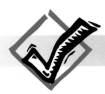

Chronic Illness Crossword Puzzle
ANSWER KEY

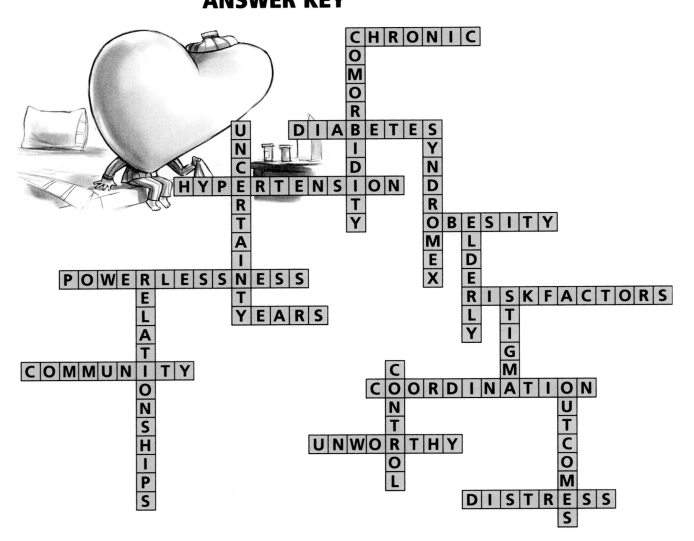

Across

1. Chronic
3. Diabetes
5. Hypertension
6. Obesity
8. Powerlessness
10. Risk factors
12. Years
13. Community
15. Coordination
17. Unworthy
18. Distress

Down

1. Comorbidity
2. Uncertainty
4. Syndrome X
7. Elderly
9. Relationships
11. Stigma
14. Control
16. Outcomes

Common Discomforts of Pregnancy Pictures

Chris Reid, RN, MSN
Bernadette Price, RN, MSN

10 to 30 minutes

Preparation

1. Copy the Discomforts of Pregnancy page.
2. Cut the page on the lines or copy them onto index cards.
3. Place strips of paper or cards into a bag.
4. Obtain flipchart or white board and appropriate markers for drawing.
5. Set the clock or stopwatch for 1 minute.

Implementation

1. Divide group into teams of equal numbers.
2. Explain the goal is to guess which discomfort is being drawn and give the correct nursing intervention or teaching.
3. Team members take turns selecting a discomfort card and illustrating it.
4. One team member begins by selecting a discomfort card. He or she tries to draw something to make his or her team read the discomfort aloud. No talking is allowed between the person drawing and the team, and only 1 minute is given.
5. Once the discomfort is correctly guessed, the team must identify the correct nursing and medical interventions and teachings.
6. The team with the most points wins.
7. Distribute prizes to winning team members.

Tool box
- Flipchart or white board
- Markers
- One of the symptoms on the Discomforts of Pregnancy page
- Bag for picking strips or cards
- Clock or stopwatch
- Small prizes

Internet/intranet variation

Scan pictures onto your computer and ask e-learners to try to guess what each picture illustrates as reinforcement of obstetric content.

Educator secrets
Learners have fun and review important concepts about pregnancy.

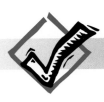

Common Discomforts of Pregnancy

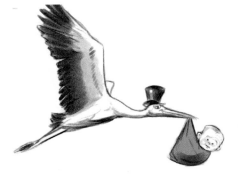

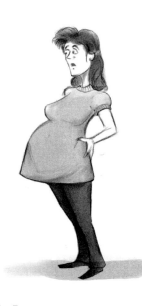

Palmer erythema

Nasal stuffiness

Backache

Leg cramps

Breast changes
(enlargement, nipple
changes)

Constipation

Pyrosis

Morning sickness   Gingivitis

Leukorrhea   Carpal tunnel

Colasma   Linea nigra

Urinary frequency   Varicosities

Mood swings   Hemorrhoids

Food cravings   Fatigue

Heart palpitations   Edema

Vena cava syndrome   Insomnia

Headache   Stria

Ptyalism   Syncope

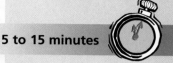

Sterile Security Patrol

Chris Reid, RN, MSN

5 to 15 minutes

Preparation

1. Obtain supplies listed in the Tool Box.

Implementation

1. Distribute the Sterile Security Patrol (SSP) badges, whistles, and tickets to selected instructors who will monitor sterile procedures performed by the demonstrators.
2. SSP officers will blow their whistles when the demonstrating students commit a breach of sterile technique.
3. Tickets naming the violation will be issued for sterile technique offenses.
4. To clear the violation, the student must be able to identify the sterile technique error and demonstrate proper sterile technique for the procedure.
5. Students consistently demonstrating proper sterile technique will earn their SSP badges. This allows them to serve on the SSP team and monitor sterile technique for other students hoping to achieve their SSP badges.
6. SSP members continue to monitor for sterile technique offenders and issue citations accordingly.
7. The goal is for all students to become members of the SSP.

Tool box
- SSP badges (can be name tags)
- One whistle per patrol member
- Various sterile procedure setups
- Tickets (or index cards) to ticket or record violations
- Instructors

Educator secrets
The instructors are the highest authority if a question of technique occurs. Students serving as SSP officers are continually reviewing their sterile technique while they monitor others.

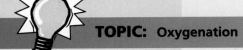
Oxygenation Word Scramble

Chris Reid, RN, MSN
Bernadette Price, RN, MSN

5 to 10 minutes

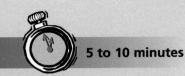

Tool box

- **One copy of the Oxygenation Word Scramble per learner**
- **One pen or pencil for each participant**
- **Oxygenation Word Scramble Answer Key**
- **Small prize**

Preparation

1. Copy the Oxygenation Word Scramble.
2. Copy the Oxygenation Word Scramble Answer Key.

Implementation

1. Distribute the Oxygenation Word Scramble, one per student.
2. Distribute a pen or pencil to each learner.
3. Explain the object of the activity is to unscramble the word using the clue given.
4. You might set a time limit, such as most correct answers in 5 minutes.
5. When time is up, share the answer key with the learners.
6. The student with the most correct answers wins a small prize.

Educator secrets

This scramble can be used to introduce or reinforce the topic. You can also use it as a quiz if you assign pre-reading on the topic before class.

Internet/intranet variation

Include this word search puzzle on-line in a course as a review opportunity.

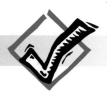

Oxygenation Word Scramble

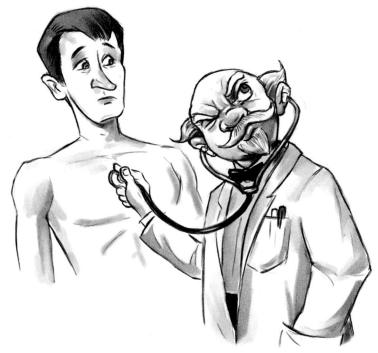

lnaunc _____	Tube on a tracheostomy
ntet _____	Method of giving oxygen
ohyxaip _____	Condition caused by lack of O_2
tchrteamyoso _____	Alternate airway
eirf _____	A danger during O_2 therapy
iwyara _____	Must be open to maintain oxygenation
saanl _____	Oxygen administration per nose
rlite _____	Measurement of oxygen flow rate
lsereti _____	Suctioning of a trach is this type of procedure
itnretinemtn _____	Type of suctioning used for tracheostomy
smak _____	Another way of administering O_2
lwaiwtarhd _____	When to apply suction with tracheostomy care upon _____
ehtyapleirtvne _____	Should be done before inserting suction catheter into tracheostomy
mesi-froewl _____	Best position for patient receiving oxygen
cciyatano _____	Color describing patient with decreased oxygen
OSB _____	Abbreviation for shortness of breath

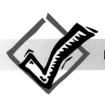

Oxygenation Word Scramble
ANSWER KEY

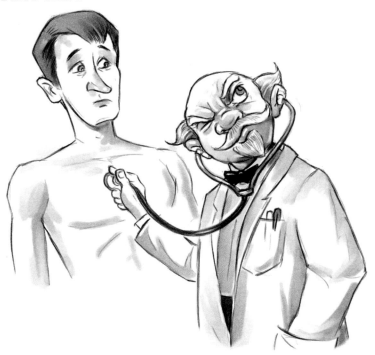

Tube on a tracheostomy—**cannula**
Method of giving oxygen—**tent**
Condition caused by lack of O₂—**hypoxia**
Alternate airway—**tracheostomy**
A danger during O₂ therapy—**fire**
Must be open to maintain oxygenation—**airway**
Oxygen administration per nose—**nasal**
Measurement of oxygen flow rate—**liter**
Suctioning of a trach is this type of procedure—**sterile**
Type of suctioning used for tracheostomy—**intermittent**
Another way of administering O₂—**mask**
Apply suction with tracheostomy care upon—**withdrawal**
Should be done before inserting suction catheter into
     tracheostomy—**hyperventilate**
Best position for patient receiving oxygen—**semi-Fowlers**
Color describing patient with decreased oxygen—**cyanotic**
Abbreviation for shortness of breath—**SOB**

Diabetes Mellitus Word Search

Margaret O'Hara, RN, MSN

15 to 30 minutes

Preparation

1. Make a copy of the Diabetes Mellitus Word Search for each participant.
2. Use this as introduction to the lesson or review after the lesson.
3. Make sure all participants have a pen or pencil.
4. Make a copy of the answer key.

Implementation

1. Distribute the Diabetes Mellitus Word Search.
2. Challenge your learners to complete the puzzle as individuals or as teams.
3. If energy and attention are low during your lesson presentation, stop and let your participants engage in this energizing activity.
4. Word search puzzles can act as pre- or posttests, and they can also be sent out days or weeks after the lesson as reinforcement of important concepts.

Variation

1. Use a poster printer copy machine to turn the word search puzzle into a poster-sized image.
2. Plan for groups of two to six to discuss and fill in a poster-sized copy of the puzzle before or after your lesson.

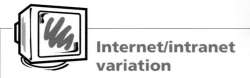

Internet/intranet variation

Include this word search puzzle on-line in a course as a review opportunity.

Tool box
- **Diabetes Mellitus Word Search**
- **Diabetes Mellitus Word Search Answer Key**
- **One pen or pencil per participant**

Educator secrets

If learners are of different ability levels in your session, pair those at different levels to maximize benefits to all participants.

141

Diabetes Mellitus Word Search

DIRECTIONS: Using the following clues, find the answers in the word search puzzle on page 144. The answers may be found vertically, horizontally, diagonally, or backward. Good luck!

1. Insulin is made in the _____ cells of the pancreas.
2. A possible causative factor of diabetes because of the antibodies is a _____.
3. Increased thirst is known as _____.
4. NPH is an _____ -acting insulin.
5. An early intervention for hypoglycemia is _____.
6. Infection and stress both _____ blood sugar.
7. Type I diabetes is also known as _____.
8. Diabetics use an _____ list to choose foods daily.
9. Human insulin is made from _____ bacteria.
10. A person who is allergic to _____ drugs should not take oral hypoglycemic agents.
11. A diabetic person should do exercise on a _____ basis.
12. CRF develops because of changes in the _____ of the kidney.
13. A diabetic person with poor circulation and poor wound healing is in _____ nitrogen balance.
14. Type II diabetes is usually a _____ onset.
15. Oral hypoglycemic agents _____ beta cells to secrete more insulin.
16. The only type of insulin that can be given by the intravenous (IV) route is _____.
17. Insulin converts glucose to _____ in muscles.
18. If no carbohydrate (CHO) is available for energy, the body uses _____.
19. Blood work drawn after meals is called _____.

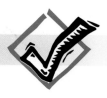

20. Increased hunger is called _____.
21. The method used by glucose to get into cells is _____.
22. Hypoglycemia is also known as _____.
23. The term for peripheral nerve degeneration is _____.
24. A steroid medication that induces diabetes is _____.
25. A special blood and urine test to diagnose diabetes mellitus is _____.
26. Insulin _____ circulating blood glucose.
27. Increased acids in the body from the breakdown of fats is known as _____.
28. A term for glucose in the urine is _____.
29. Three things necessary for the treatment of diabetes are _____, _____, and _____.
30. Strenuous exercise during peak insulin time should be avoided to prevent _____.
31. Polyuria is increased _____.
32. Atrophy of tissues caused by repeated injections of cold insulin in the same spot is called _____.
33. PZI is a _____-acting insulin.
34. Mixing of insulin is done from _____ to _____.
35. The abbreviation for diabetic ketoacidosis is _____.
36. Deep gasping of a person in diabetic ketoacidosis is known as _____ respirations.
37. The characteristic "fruity" odor is found in a person with a complication of _____.
38. _____ refers to regular insulin given in response to glucose monitoring three to four times a day.
39. Continuous regular insulin infusion may be given via a _____.
40. The response of a person to treatment of hypoglycemia is usually _____.

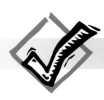

Diabetes Mellitus Word Search—cont'd

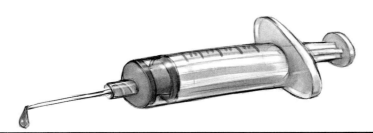

R	E	X	E	R	C	I	S	E	H	K	A	M	D	D	I	N	K
O	H	Y	P	E	R	G	L	Y	C	E	M	I	A	E	N	P	U
U	Y	E	C	G	G	E	S	A	A	T	E	B	I	L	T	M	S
T	H	A	O	U	L	N	T	I	N	O	D	S	M	A	E	U	S
I	P	M	N	L	Y	I	I	R	D	A	I	E	E	C	R	P	M
N	O	F	R	A	C	R	M	U	Y	C	C	S	C	S	M	O	A
E	R	S	A	R	O	U	U	S	D	I	A	A	Y	G	E	L	U
G	T	U	P	T	G	Y	L	O	U	D	T	E	L	N	D	Y	L
N	S	R	I	R	E	U	A	C	O	O	I	R	G	I	I	P	O
A	Y	I	D	O	N	F	T	Y	L	S	O	C	O	D	A	H	N
H	D	V	I	A	L	I	E	L	C	I	N	E	P	I	T	A	G
C	O	L	A	U	D	A	R	G	O	S	S	D	Y	L	E	G	L
X	P	O	S	T	P	R	A	N	D	I	A	L	H	S	N	I	O
E	I	T	R	O	P	S	N	A	R	T	E	V	I	T	C	A	M
G	L	U	C	O	S	E	T	O	L	E	R	A	N	C	E	T	E
I	N	C	R	E	A	S	E	N	O	S	I	N	D	E	R	P	R
P	O	L	Y	D	I	P	S	I	A	E	C	O	L	I	D	I	U
U	S	E	D	K	M	O	Y	H	T	A	P	O	R	U	E	N	L
I	T	A	W	A	D	D	I	N	E	G	A	T	I	V	E	T	U
M	A	R	T	S	K	C	O	H	S	N	I	L	U	S	N	I	S

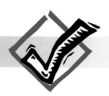

Diabetes Mellitus Word Search
ANSWERS

1. Insulin is made in the **beta** cells of the pancreas.
2. A possible causative factor of diabetes because of the antibodies is a **virus.**
3. Increased thirst is known as **polydipsia.**
4. NPH is an **intermediate**-acting insulin.
5. An early intervention for hypoglycemia is **candy.**
6. Infection and stress both **increase** blood sugar.
7. Type I diabetes is also known as **IDDM.**
8. Diabetics use an **exchange** list to choose foods daily.
9. Human insulin is made from **E. coli** bacteria.
10. A person who is allergic to **sulfa** drugs should not take oral hypoglycemic agents.
11. A diabetic person should do exercise on a **routine** basis.
12. CRF develops because of changes in the **glomerulus** of the kidney.
13. A diabetic person with poor circulation and poor wound healing is in **negative** nitrogen balance.
14. Type II diabetes is usually a **gradual** onset.
15. Oral hypoglycemic agents **stimulate** beta cells to secrete more insulin.
16. The only type of insulin that can be given by the IV route is **regular.**
17. Insulin converts glucose to **glycogen** in muscles.
18. If no CHO is available for energy, the body uses **fat.**
19. Blood work drawn after meals is called **postprandial.**

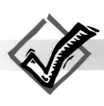

Diabetes Mellitus Word Search
ANSWERS—cont'd

20. Increased hunger is called **polyphagia.**
21. The method used by glucose to get into cells is **active transport.**
22. Hypoglycemia is also known as **insulin shock.**
23. The term for peripheral nerve degeneration is **neuropathy.**
24. A steroid medication that induces diabetes is **prednisone.**
25. A special blood and urine test to diagnose diabetes mellitus is **glucose tolerance.**
26. Insulin **decreases** circulating blood glucose.
27. Increased acids in the body from the breakdown of fats is known as **ketoacidosis.**
28. A term for glucose in the urine is **glycosuria.**
29. Three things necessary for the treatment of diabetes are **diet, exercise,** and **medications.**
30. Strenuous exercise during peak insulin time should be avoided to prevent **hypoglycemia.**
31. Polyuria is increased **urine.**
32. Atrophy of tissues caused by repeated injections of cold insulin in the same spot is called **lipodystrophy.**
33. PZI is a **long**-acting insulin.
34. Mixing of insulin is done from **clear** to **cloudy.**
35. The abbreviation for diabetic ketoacidosis is **DKA.**
36. Deep gasping of a person in diabetic ketoacidosis is known as **Kussmaul** respirations.
37. The characteristic "fruity" odor is found in a person with a complication of **hyperglycemia.**
38. **Sliding scale** refers to regular insulin given in response to glucose monitoring three to four times a day.
39. Continuous regular insulin infusion may be given via a **pump.**
40. The response of a person to treatment of hypoglycemia is usually **rapid.**

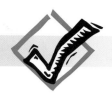

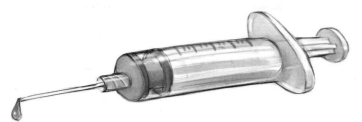

```
R  E  X  E  R  C  I  S  E  H  K  A  M  D  D  I  N  K
O  H  Y  P  E  R  G  L  Y  C  E  M  I  A  E  N  P  U
U  Y  E  C  G  G  E  S  A  A  T  E  B  I  L  T  M  S
T  H  A  O  U  L  N  T  I  N  O  D  S  M  A  E  U  S
I  P  M  N  L  Y  I  I  R  D  A  I  E  E  C  R  P  M
N  O  F  R  A  C  R  M  U  Y  C  C  S  C  S  M  O  A
E  R  S  A  R  O  U  U  S  D  A  A  C  Y  E  E  L  U
G  T  U  P  T  G  Y  L  O  U  D  T  A  L  G  D  Y  L
N  S  R  I  R  E  Y  U  C  O  O  I  E  R  N  I  P  O
A  Y  I  D  O  N  F  L  O  S  O  C  G  O  D  A  H  N
H  D  V  I  A  L  U  A  L  C  S  E  I  D  A  T  A  G
C  O  L  A  U  D  A  R  G  I  N  S  D  I  E  G  I  L
X  P  O  S  T  P  R  A  N  D  I  A  L  H  S  N  I  O
E  I  T  R  O  P  S  N  A  R  T  E  V  I  T  C  A  M
G  L  U  C  O  S  E  T  O  L  E  R  A  N  C  E  T  E
I  N  C  R  E  A  S  E  N  O  S  I  N  D  E  R  P  R
P  O  L  Y  D  I  P  S  I  A  E  C  O  L  I  D  I  U
U  S  E  D  K  M  O  Y  H  T  A  P  O  R  U  E  N  L
I  T  A  W  A  D  D  I  N  E  G  A  T  I  V  E  T  U
M  A  R  T  S  K  C  O  H  S  N  I  L  U  S  N  I  S
```

TOPIC: Labor and birth information

Labor and Birth Questions, Not Answers

20 to 30 minutes   Bernadette Price, MSN, RN

Tool box
- **Game board with categories and point amounts on overhead transparency (projector), PowerPoint screens (computer and display setup), or posters**
- **Answer sheets**
- **Question sheet**
- **Buzzing device**
- **Self-adhesive notes**
- **Watch with a second hand or timing device**
- **Variety of small prizes**

Educator secrets
Create a fun atmosphere, and equalize participation as much as possible.

Preparation

1. Review the information on the ready-to-use answer sheet and questions sheet and make any adaptations necessary to your facility.
2. Create a projectable image of the amount and category sheet. (An overhead transparency, PowerPoint screen, or even a poster will do.)
3. Copy the answer sheet for yourself. This is for you to read to the learners when they pick a category and an amount.
4. Make a copy of the answer key questions. This is for you to check your learners' responses to see if they are correct.
5. Obtain a buzzing device to determine which team rings in first.
6. Place self-adhesive notes on the category and amount transparency or poster squares after they have been chosen. Place an "X" over PowerPoint squares. This will make it easy for the learners to see what can still be chosen.
7. Collect a variety of small prizes or goodies (fruit, stickers, pins, pens) to award to participants at the end of the activity.

Implementation

1. Divide the group into two or more teams of three to six learners.
2. Explain that the teams may collaborate before answering the question.
3. Present the categories:
   a. It's Never Too Late has to do with early labor.
   b. Be Actively Involved is focused on active labor.
   c. Shut Up, I'm in a crisis! is about transition.
   d. You're a Pain in the Butt! is about pain relief measures.
   e. The "I"s Have It is a category in which every answer begins with the letter "I."
4. Select a team to go first. Display the playing board. A spokesperson for the group selects a category and an amount.
5. The instructor reads the answer from that category and the amount.

148

6. The teams can discuss their ideas quietly for up to 5 seconds before answering.

7. A team representative states the question that fits the answer the instructor has given.

8. If the question given is correct, the team is awarded points based on how much their question was worth. If the answer is incorrect, the instructor can give the other teams a chance to answer or simply reveal the correct answer. If the question has an asterisk by it, the team can wager as many points as they might have.

9. Points are tallied for each team.

10. After all answers are given, the team with the most points wins.

11. Prizes are awarded to all participants, with those with the highest points selecting their gifts first. Because their knowledge has increased, they are all winners.

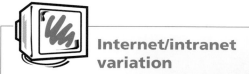

Internet/intranet variation

This can be used as a pretest or posttest or review in an Internet course.

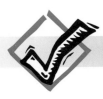

Labor and Birth Questions, Not Answers
AMOUNT AND CATEGORY SHEET

DIRECTIONS: This playing board can be made into a projectable visual or a poster.

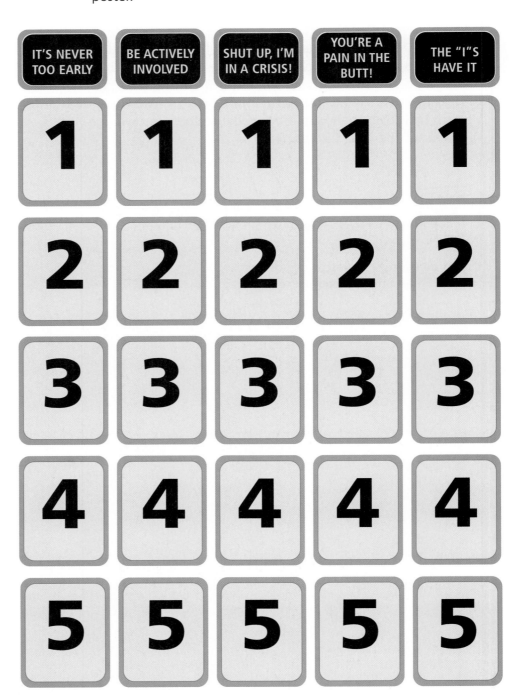

IT'S NEVER TOO EARLY	BE ACTIVELY INVOLVED	SHUT UP, I'M IN A CRISIS!	YOU'RE A PAIN IN THE BUTT!	THE "I"S HAVE IT
1	1	1	1	1
2	2	2	2	2
3	3	3	3	3
4	4	4	4	4
5	5	5	5	5

150

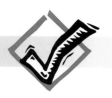

Labor and Birth Questions, Not Answers
ANSWERS

DIRECTIONS: This playing board can be made into an overhead transparency or downloaded into PowerPoint.

IT'S NEVER TOO EARLY	BE ACTIVELY INVOLVED	SHUT UP, I'M IN A CRISIS!	YOU'RE A PAIN IN THE BUTT!	THE "I"S HAVE IT
This is the shortening of the longitudinal muscles of the uterus.	By definition, this is the amount of cervical dilation occurring in the active phase of labor.	This is the breathing technique used during an urge to push. It is also useful when making a wish on birthday.	This is a narcotic antagonist.	This is a complication of prolonged ruptured membranes.
This is a sanguineous discharge.	A woman in active labor or an obscene phone caller might breathe like this. (Please demonstrate.)	This is a mood change commonly displayed by a woman in transition.	This is the potential concern of giving a narcotic before active labor is established.	Rapid breathing may lead to a fluid volume deficit of this.
"Don't drop me, Mom," might be what a fetus says when this premonitory sign of labor occurs.	If the woman tells her partner that labor has become a "tingling experience," you might suspect this is happening.	This may not be earth shaking, but it certainly is a bed-shaking experience (seen in the woman in transition).	This position will help correct hypotension after an epidural.	This is the part of the pelvis used in identifying station.
Robins do this in the spring (so do some women before labor begins).	A woman in active labor might lose this. If a clown lost this, he or she would be out of a job.	This is a safe place to be (often expressed by a woman in transition). Dorothy and Toto wanted to go there too.	This is a regional anesthesia that is injected for an episiotomy repair.	These are two methods used to administer medication to the laboring woman.
As a high school senior, you may have attended this special dance (as a mom starting labor, you might find this a fluid-filled experience).	These are the three positions that can facilitate labor progression.	These are three stomach upsets that might occur during transition.	If a medication causes hypotension in mom, it will lead to this adverse effect in the baby.	This defect in the fetus may cause hydramnios.

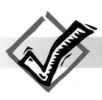

Labor and Birth Questions, Not Answers
ANSWER KEY QUESTIONS

DIRECTIONS: This playing board can be made into an overhead transparency, downloaded into PowerPoint, or used as your answer key copied on paper. The learner should place his or her answer in the form of a question, as shown following.

IT'S NEVER TOO EARLY	BE ACTIVELY INVOLVED	SHUT UP, I'M IN A CRISIS!	YOU'RE A PAIN IN THE BUTT!	THE "I"S HAVE IT
What is a contraction?	What is 3 to 8 cm?	What is blowing?	What is Narcan?	What is an infection?
What is bloody show discharge?	What is shallow or modified paced breathing?	What is irritable or withdrawn?	What is slow-stop labor?	What is insensible water loss?
What is lightening?	What is hyper-ventilation?	What is trembling?	What is lateral?	What are the ischial spines?
What is nesting?	What is a sense of humor?	What is home?	What is a local or pudendal?	What is IM and IV?
What is P.R.O.M?	What is squat, stand, sit, hands-knees walk?	What is N&V, burping, heartburn, hiccoughs?	What is hypoxia?	What is imperforated anus?

GI Disorders Word Search

Margaret O'Hara, RN, MSN

15 to 30 minutes

Preparation

1. Make a copy of the ready-to-use gastrointestinal (GI) Disorders Word Search for each participant.
2. Use this as introduction to the lesson or review after the lesson.
3. Make sure all participants have a pen or pencil.
4. Make a copy of the answer key.

> **Tool box**
> - GI Disorders Word Search
> - GI Disorders Word Search Answer Key
> - One pen or pencil per participant

Implementation

1. Distribute the large or small GI Disorders Word Search.
2. Challenge your learners to complete the puzzle as individuals or as teams.
3. If energy and attention are low during your lesson presentation, stop and let your participants engage in this energizing activity.
4. Word search puzzles can act as pretests or posttests, and they can also be sent out days or weeks after the lesson as reinforcement of important concepts.

Variation

1. Use a poster printer copy machine to turn the word search puzzle into a poster-sized image.
2. Plan for groups of two to six to discuss and fill in a poster-sized copy of the puzzle before or after your lesson.

> **Educator secrets**
> If you have different ability levels in your session, pair learners to maximize benefits to all participants.

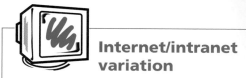

> **Internet/intranet variation**
> Include this word search puzzle on-line in a course as a review opportunity.

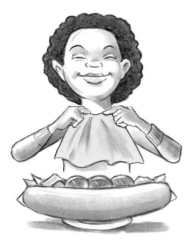

GI Disorders Word Search

DIRECTIONS: Using the following clues, find the answers in the word search
Puzzle on the facing page. The answer may be found vertically,
horizontally, diagonally, or backward. Good luck!

1. Looking into various areas of the body by using a flexible instrument is called an _____.
2. A radiograph that gives information about the chemical makeup of tissues is an _____.
3. A test for occult blood is called _____.
4. Aspiration of fluid from the peritoneal cavity is called a _____.
5. Kidneys convert ammonia to _____.
6. After a liver biopsy, turn the patient to the _____.
7. Vomiting of blood is known as _____.
8. A term for a large amount of fat in the stool is _____.
9. An inflammatory disorder of the lining of the stomach is _____.
10. Bile is produced by the _____.
11. Common obstruction that causes cholecystitis is called _____.
12. Acute pancreatitis causes severe abdominal pain radiating to the _____.
13. A term used to describe vomitus with old blood in it is _____.
14. The opening in the diaphragm where the esophagus meets the stomach is the _____.
15. Enlarging the pyloric sphincter to enhance gastric emptying is a _____.
16. A test to view the stomach mucosa is _____.
17. A digestive enzyme produced by the pancreas for fat breakdown is _____.
18. An ulcer involving areas of the GI tract is a _____ ulcer.
19. An endoscopic retrograde cholangiopancreatography examination is commonly called _____.
20. This drug is considered a mucosal fortifier and is called _____.
21. A complication after a gastrectomy in which food rapidly enters the small intestine is called _____.
22. Common name of the tube inserted into a bile duct for drainage is a _____.
23. Yellow coloration of the skin and the whites of eyes is known as _____.

154

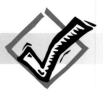

GI Disorders Word Search

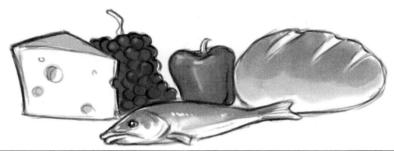

```
B  I  L  S  T  E  A  T  O  R  R  H  E  A  D
A  E  R  U  V  A  G  O  T  O  M  Y  S  F  U
D  N  U  O  R  G  E  E  F  F  O  C  U  A  M
A  D  G  A  S  T  R  O  S  C  O  P  Y  T  P
C  O  J  A  U  N  D  I  C  E  N  R  L  T  I
H  S  I  S  E  M  E  T  A  M  E  H  E  Y  N
I  C  E  R  C  P  B  A  C  K  D  A  F  C  G
A  O  S  E  N  O  T  S  A  Y  I  N  T  A  S
T  P  A  R  A  C  E  N  T  E  S  I  S  R  Y
U  Y  C  L  A  W  I  S  M  T  T  R  I  A  N
S  I  T  I  R  T  S  A  G  T  H  M  D  F  D
I  M  A  T  T  E  O  A  I  U  G  H  E  A  R
N  U  N  I  A  P  V  N  C  B  I  D  O  T  O
G  L  I  P  A  S  E  I  B  E  R  T  H  E  M
P  P  Y  L  O  R  O  P  L  A  S  T  Y  S  E
```

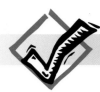

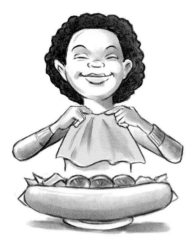

GI Disorders Word Search
ANSWERS

1. Looking into various areas of the body by using a flexible instrument is called an **endoscopy.**
2. A radiograph that gives information about the chemical makeup of tissues is an **MRI.**
3. A test for occult blood is called **guaiac.**
4. Aspiration of fluid from the peritoneal cavity is called a **paracentesis.**
5. Kidneys convert ammonia to **urea.**
6. After a liver biopsy, turn the patient to the **right side.**
7. Vomiting of blood is known as **hematemesis.**
8. A term for a large amount of fat in the stool is **steatorrhea.**
9. An inflammatory disorder of the lining of the stomach is **gastritis.**
10. Bile is produced by the **liver.**
11. Common obstruction that causes cholecystitis is called **stones.**
12. Acute pancreatitis causes severe abdominal pain radiating to the **back.**
13. A term used to describe vomitus with old blood in it is **coffee grounds.**
14. The opening in the diaphragm where the esophagus meets the stomach is the **hiatus.**
15. Enlarging the pyloric sphincter to enhance gastric emptying is a **pyloroplasty.**
16. A test to view the stomach mucosa is **gastroscopy.**
17. A digestive enzyme produced by the pancreas for fat breakdown is **lipase.**
18. A type of ulcer involving areas of the GI tract is a **peptic** ulcer.
19. An endoscopic retrograde cholangiopancreatography examination is commonly called **ERCP.**
20. This drug is considered a mucosal fortifier and is called **Carafate.**
21. A complication after a gastrectomy in which food rapidly enters the small intestine is called **dumping syndrome.**
22. Common name of the tube inserted into a bile duct for drainage is a **T tube.**
23. Yellow coloration of the skin and the whites of eyes is known as **jaundice.**

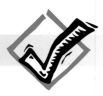

GI Disorders Word Search
ANSWER KEY

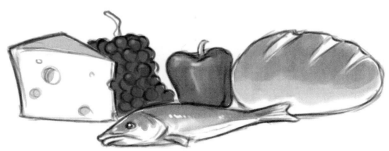

B	I	L	L	S	T	E	A	T	O	R	R	H	E	A	D
A	E	R	U	V	A	G	O	T	O	M	Y	S	F	U
D	N	U	O	R	G	E	E	F	F	O	C	U	A	M
A	D	G	A	S	T	R	O	S	C	O	P	Y	T	P
C	O	J	A	U	N	D	I	C	E	N	R	L	T	I
H	S	I	S	E	M	E	T	A	M	E	H	E	Y	N
I	C	E	R	C	P	B	A	C	K	D	A	F	C	G
A	O	S	E	N	O	T	S	A	Y	I	N	T	A	S
T	P	A	R	A	C	E	N	T	E	S	I	S	R	Y
U	Y	C	L	A	W	I	S	M	T	T	R	I	A	N
S	I	T	I	R	T	S	A	G	T	H	M	D	F	D
I	M	A	T	T	E	O	A	I	U	G	H	E	A	R
N	U	N	I	A	P	V	N	C	B	I	D	O	T	O
G	L	I	P	A	S	E	I	B	E	R	T	H	E	M
P	P	Y	L	O	R	O	P	L	A	S	T	Y	S	E

CVA Word Search

Margaret O'Hara, RN, MSN

15 to 30 minutes

Tool box
- **CVA Word Search**
- **CVA Word Search Answer Key**
- **One pen or pencil per participant**

Preparation

1. Make a copy of the ready-to-use cerebral vascular accident (CVA) Word Search for each participant.
2. Use this as an introduction to the lesson or review after the lesson.
3. Make sure all participants have a pen or pencil.
4. Make a copy of the answer key.

Implementation

1. Distribute the large or small CVA Word Search.
2. Challenge your learners to complete the puzzle as individuals or as teams.
3. If energy and attention are low during your lesson presentation, stop and let your participants engage in this energizing activity.
4. Word search puzzles can act as pretest or posttests, and they can also be sent out days or weeks after the lesson as reinforcement of important concepts.

Variation

1. Use a poster printer copy machine to turn the word search puzzle into a poster-sized image.
2. Plan for groups of two to six to discuss and fill in a poster-sized copy of the puzzle before or after your lesson.

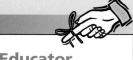

Educator secrets
If you have different ability levels in your session, pair learners to maximize benefits to all participants.

Internet/intranet variation
Include this word search puzzle on-line in a course as a review opportunity.

158

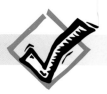

CVA Word Search

DIRECTIONS: Using the following clues, find the answers in the Word Search
Puzzle on page 159. The answers may be found vertically, horizontally, diagonally, or backward. Good luck!

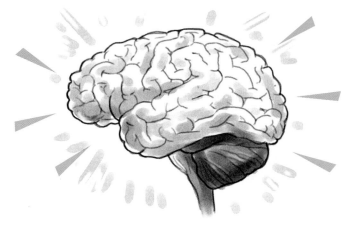

1. Broca's speech is located in the _____ of the brain.
2. A problem in the cerebrum will present signs and symptoms on
   the _____ side of the body.
3. Communication between the carotid arteries and the vertebral
   arteries is known as the _____.
4. Denial of a body part can lead to _____ of that
   part.
5. A stationary blood clot is called a _____.
6. A major function of the brain stem is to help regulate
   _____.
7. A separation or dislocation of joint surfaces is called
   _____.
8. The _____ lobe of the brain controls visual images
   of the past.
9. Temporary impairment of neurologic functioning without permanent damage is called _____.
10. Damage usually occurs suddenly in a stroke caused from a
    _____.
11. A test for coordination and balance is the _____
    test.
12. A procedure done to remove plaque from carotid arteries is called
    a carotid _____.
13. Loss of ability to recognize size, shape, and texture of objects is
    called _____.

Continued

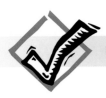

CVA Word Search—cont'd

14. Wernicke's speech is located in the _____ lobe of the brain.
15. Paralysis or weakness of oral muscles necessary for articulation of speech is called _____.
16. Constant repetition of a phrase or activity is known as

    _____.
17. _____ is paralysis of voluntary muscles on one side of the body.
18. The cerebellum controls coordination and _____.
19. Broca's speech is also known as _____ speech.
20. The _____ lobe is the principle sensory area of the brain.
21. Lack of coordination is called _____.
22. A client who has had a right CVA and left hemiparesis usually has a problem with _____.
23. A permanent neurologic deficit with no further progression is called a _____ stroke.
24. A problem in the cerebellum will present signs and symptoms on the _____ side of the body.
25. The prefrontal lobe of the brain controls _____ and

    _____.
26. Wernicke's speech is also known as _____ speech.
27. The term used for knowing where body parts are in space without looking at them is _____.
28. Two important areas of the brain stem are the
    _____ and the _____.
29. The speech areas of the brain are usually found on the
    _____ side of the brain.
30. Blindness in half the field of vision in one or two eyes is called

    _____.
31. Loss of ability to carry out a previously learned activity is called

    _____.
32. Paralysis of muscles used in swallowing is _____.
33. _____ is weakness on one side of the body.
34. A third name describing Wernicke's aphasia is

    _____.
35. _____ nerve tracts cross over in the lower edge of the medulla.
36. An intervention to reinforce with a client with hemianopsia is

    _____.
37. With the problem of dysphagia, a nursing goal would be to prevent _____.

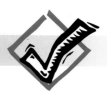

CVA Word Search

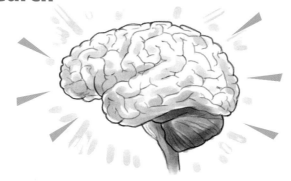

C	O	M	P	L	E	T	E	D	Y	S	A	R	T	H	R	I	A
H	P	R	O	P	R	I	O	C	E	P	T	I	O	N	K	E	H
O	E	O	P	P	O	S	I	T	E	B	C	M	P	O	L	N	E
S	R	F	N	E	A	I	G	A	H	P	S	Y	D	I	A	D	M
A	S	G	I	S	W	Y	D	T	B	R	O	C	A	T	T	A	I
F	E	K	A	H	E	M	I	A	N	O	P	S	I	A	I	R	P
E	V	M	H	L	C	A	B	X	C	H	A	R	N	X	P	T	A
T	E	X	P	R	E	S	S	I	V	E	O	D	A	U	I	E	R
Y	R	A	P	H	A	S	I	A	A	T	G	R	F	L	C	R	E
T	A	S	P	I	R	A	T	I	O	N	P	H	E	B	C	E	S
I	T	L	A	M	S	W	X	M	C	A	O	F	I	U	O	C	I
L	I	B	R	A	I	N	B	R	P	S	T	N	F	S	U	T	S
A	O	C	I	R	C	L	E	O	F	W	I	L	L	I	S	O	H
N	N	V	E	Q	U	I	T	M	R	A	L	L	U	D	E	M	A
O	U	Y	T	H	R	O	M	B	U	S	D	F	E	V	A	Y	I
S	P	B	A	L	A	N	C	E	W	E	R	N	N	I	P	G	S
R	O	T	L	A	T	N	O	R	F	C	L	O	T	W	H	I	O
E	H	E	M	I	P	L	E	G	I	A	T	C	E	L	G	E	N
P	V	I	T	A	L	S	I	G	N	S	C	A	N	N	I	N	G
S	J	U	D	G	M	E	N	T	E	M	P	O	R	A	L	L	A
H	E	M	O	R	R	H	A	G	E	V	I	T	P	E	C	E	R

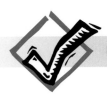

CVA Word Search
ANSWERS

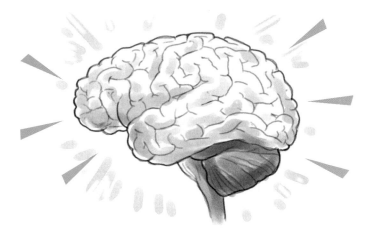

1. Broca's speech is located in the **frontal** area of the brain.
2. A problem in the cerebrum will present signs and symptoms on the **opposite** side of the body.
3. Communication between the carotid arteries and the vertebral arteries is known as the **circle of Willis.**
4. Denial of a body part can lead to **neglect** of that part.
5. A stationary blood clot is called a **thrombus.**
6. A major function of the brain stem is to help regulate **vital signs.**
7. A separation or dislocation of joint surfaces is called **subluxation.**
8. The **occipital** lobe of the brain controls visual images of the past.
9. Temporary impairment of neurologic functioning without permanent damage is called **TIA.**
10. Damage usually occurs suddenly in a stroke caused from a **hemorrhage.**
11. A test for coordination and balance is the **Romberg** test.
12. A procedure done to remove plaque from carotid arteries is called a carotid **endarterectomy.**
13. Loss of ability to recognize size, shape, and texture of objects is called **agnosia.**
14. Wernicke's speech is located in the **temporal** lobe of the brain.
15. Paralysis or weakness of oral muscles necessary for articulation of speech is called **dysarthria.**

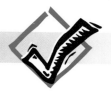

16. Constant repetition of a phrase or activity is known as **perseveration.**
17. **Hemiplegia** is paralysis of voluntary muscles on one side of the body.
18. The cerebellum controls coordination and **balance.**
19. Broca's speech is also known as **expressive** speech.
20. The **parietal** lobe is the principle sensory area of the brain.
21. Lack of coordination is called **ataxia.**
22. A client who has had a right CVA and left hemiparesis usually has a problem with **safety.**
23. Permanent neurologic deficit with no further progression is called a **completed** stroke.
24. A problem in the cerebellum will present signs and symptoms on the **same** side of the body.
25. The prefrontal lobe of the brain controls **personality** and **judgment.**
26. Wernicke's speech is also known as **receptive** speech.
27. The term used for knowing where body parts are in space without looking at them is **proprioception.**
28. Two important areas of the brain stem are the **pons** and the **medulla.**
29. The speech areas of the brain are usually found on the **left** side of the brain.
30. Blindness in half the field of vision in one or two eyes is called **hemianopsia.**
31. Loss of ability to carry out a previously learned activity is called **apraxia.**
32. Paralysis of muscles used in swallowing is **dysphagia.**
33. **Hemiparesis** is weakness on one side of the body.
34. A third name describing Wernicke's aphasia is **fluent.**
35. **Motor** nerve tracts cross over in the lower edge of the medulla.
36. An intervention to reinforce with a client with hemianopsia is **scanning.**
37. With the problem of dysphagia, a nursing goal would be to prevent **aspiration.**

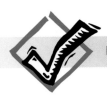

CVA Word Search
ANSWER KEY

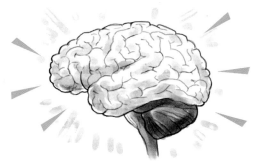

```
C O M P L E T E D Y S A R T H R I A
H P R O P R I O C E P T I O N K E H
O E O P P O S I T E B C M P O L N E
S R F N E A I G A H P S Y D I A D M
A S G I S W Y D T B R O C A T T A I
F E K A H E M I A N O P S I A I R P
E V M H L C A B X C H A R N X P T A
T E X P R E S S I V E O D A U I R R
Y R A P H A S I A A T G R F L C E E
T A S P I R A T I O N P H E B C S S
I T L A M S W X M C A O F I U O I I
L I B R A I N B R P S T N F S U T S
A O C I R C L E O F W I L L I S O H
N V E Q U I T M R A L L U D E M A
O U Y T H R O M B U S D F E V A Y I
S P B A L A N C E W E R N N I P G S
R O T L A T N O R F C L O T W H I O
E H E M I P L E G I A T C E L G E N
P V I T A L S I G N S C A N N I N G
S J U D G M E N T E M P O R A L L A
H E M O R R H A G E V I T P E C E R
```

Makin' Money—Med-Surg Style

Iris Trahan, RN, BSN, CCRN

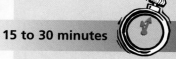

15 to 30 minutes

Preparation

1. Select a contestant who will answer the questions asked.
2. Give the participant his or her copy of the question cards.

Implementation

1. Explain that the participants are each given 1 minute from the completion of the reading of the question to give an answer.
2. The participant can use any of his or her two "Booster Shots" if he or she becomes stumped on a question. Distribute the cards to the participant to hold up at appropriate times. Once the cards are used, collect them from the contestant.
3. He or she can also pick "Divided Doses." In this case the course coordinator deletes two wrong answers, leaving only the right answer and one other choice.
4. Finally, the participant can "Needle a Friend." This option allows the contestant to choose a member of the audience to give an opinion about the correct answer. This option has a 1 minute time limit.
5. Recruit an audience member to keep track of the level of prizes on the flipchart for you.
6. The contestant continues to play until he or she earns the big prize or answers incorrectly. Another contestant can then take over in the player's chair.

Tool box

- Flip chart for scoring grid
- Timer
- Two chairs
- Laminated cards that say: Booster Shots, Needle a Friend, Divided Doses
- The Makin' Money —Med-Surg Style questions list for the participant and the question list with the answers for the host or hostess
- Master poster indicating the level achieved with a monetary value attached to each level
- Prizes based on level of achievement or confines of the budget

Continued

Makin' Money—Med-Surg Style—cont'd

Educator secrets

People like to get involved.

7. Stage a fun celebration as prizes are awarded to winners. Some sample prizes might be:
   - $1000 to $5000—pens, pencils, note pads
   - $10,000—coffee mug
   - $100,000—coffee mug, candy, and a cap
   - $250,000—small gift basket
   - $500,000—medium gift basket or American Hospital Association (AHA) pocket guide
   - $1,000,000—large gift basket or free course registration

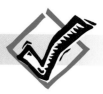

Makin' Money—Med-Surg Style Questions

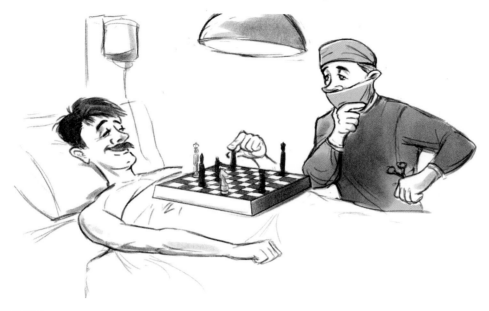

EASY

1. What can cause a change in papillary responsiveness?
   a. Pulmonary embolus
   b. Acute myocardial infarction (MI)
   c. GI bleed
   d. Brain stem lesions
2. Of the following, which situation would be least serious in the assessment of arousability?
   a. Unable to arouse
   b. Arouses to shaking
   c. Arouses to name
   d. Arouses to noxious stimuli
3. In what situation would physician notification *not* be an immediate priority?
   a. Changes in vital signs
   b. Posturing
   c. Changes in level of consciousness (LOC)
   d. Fixed and dilated pupils
4. Which of the following best describes the type of pedal pulses seen in a patient with a dissecting abdominal aortic aneurysm?
   a. Unchanged
   b. Decreased
   c. Bounding
   d. Absent

Continued

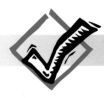

Makin' Money—Med-Surg Style
Questions—cont'd

EASY—cont'd

5. A sudden fullness in the throat followed by a rush of blood indicates which of the following?
   a. Gastritis
   b. Peptic ulcer
   c. Hemorrhoids
   d. Esophageal varices

6. The color of stools in the patient with a lower GI bleed would be which of the following?
   a. Yellow
   b. Bile colored
   c. Tarry
   d. Light brown

7. Which of the following is the location of the origin of the coronary arteries?
   a. Superior vena cava
   b. Sinoatrial (SA) node
   c. Pulmonary artery
   d. Base of the aorta

8. Shock is commonly associated in the patient with a systolic blood pressure of:
   a. 100 mm Hg
   b. 80 mm Hg
   c. 60 mm Hg
   d. 90 mm Hg

9. How does morphine relieve chest pain in the patient with an acute MI?
   a. Widens the diameter of the arteries of the heart
   b. Thins the blood where the blockage is located
   c. Increases the heart rate and blood pressure
   d. Narrows the blood vessel diameter

10. Which of the following is a common indicator of an abdominal aortic aneurysm?
   a. Hematomas or petechia
   b. Jaundice
   c. Pulsatile abdominal mass
   d. Hyperperistalsis

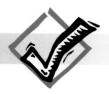

11. The normal capillary refill is how many seconds?
    a. 3 to 4
    b. 5 to 6
    c. Less than 2
    d. Less than 1

12. While replacing lost fluids, which of the following indicates fluid overload?
    a. Tarry stools
    b. Congestive heart failure (CHF)
    c. Diuresis
    d. Visual changes

13. The rhythm disturbance seen in acute MI that accounts for sudden death is which of the following?
    a. Ventricular tachycardia
    b. Complete heart block
    c. Ventricular fibrillation
    d. Atrial fibrillation

14. Angina pectoris typically radiates to which of the following?
    a. Lower abdomen
    b. Neck and jaw
    c. Flank area
    d. Back of the neck

15. How much urine does a typical adult produce per hour?
    a. 100 cc
    b. 30 cc
    c. 60 cc
    d. 45 cc

16. Angina pain typically lasts how long?
    a. Less than 1 minute
    b. 5 to 10 minutes
    c. 10 minutes or more
    d. Less than 5 minutes

17. What does *exsanguination* mean?
    a. Blockage of a coronary artery
    b. Elvis has left the building
    c. Rapid blood loss
    d. Stroke

18. How long do you wait between position changes when assessing orthostatic vital signs?
    a. 2 minutes
    b. 5 minutes
    c. 1 minute
    d. 4 minutes

Continued

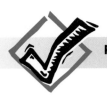

Makin' Money—Med-Surg Style
Questions—cont'd

MODERATE

1. Muffled or distant breath sounds can indicate which of the following?
   a. Cardiac tamponade
   b. Hemothorax
   c. GI bleeding
   d. You need new stethoscope

2. The patient experiencing angina usually describes the pain as:
   a. Mild-to-moderate
   b. Light
   c. Severe
   d. Excruciating

3. Which of the following is *not* a potential cause of a change in a patient's level of consciousness?
   a. Lesions of the brain
   b. Hypoxia
   c. Hemorrhage
   d. Mild-to-moderate hypoglycemia

4. Which patient position is useful for the patient with a pulmonary embolus?
   a. Trendelenburg
   b. Reverse Trendelenburg
   c. Semi-Fowler's
   d. Lying flat

5. In assessing a patient with an acute stroke, which of the following would *not* be your first priority?
   a. Speech
   b. Extremity strength
   c. Pupillary responsiveness
   d. Assessment of vital signs

6. Which of the following would *not* result in papillary size and reaction?
   a. Increased intracranial pressure (ICP)
   b. Metabolic disturbances
   c. Neurodeterioration
   d. Pulmonary embolus

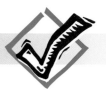

7. Which of the following can indicate fluid around the heart or pericardial tamponade?
   a. Extra heart sounds
   b. Muffled heart sounds
   c. Heart murmurs
   d. Gallop heart sounds

8. Which of the following indicates a positive finding for orthostatic systolic blood pressure changes?
   a. Drop of less than 20 mm Hg
   b. Increase of greater than 20 mm Hg
   c. Increase of 10 mm Hg
   d. Decrease of 10 mm Hg

9. An appropriate definition of hemiparesis is which of the following?
   a. Paralysis
   b. Flaccidity
   c. Weakness
   d. Lack of movement

10. Of the following, which is an early indicator of neurologic damage?
    a. Change in vital signs
    b. Posturing
    c. Changes in LOC
    d. Fixed and dilated pupils

11. Which of the following is *false* about status epilepticus?
    a. Characterized by a series of seizures
    b. Persists 20 to 30 minutes without a recovery period
    c. Usually does not require medication
    d. Is potentially life threatening

12. What percentage of emboli develop from a blood clot?
    a. 99%
    b. 90%
    c. 75%
    d. 95%

13. The assessment that indicates evaluation of level of consciousness is:
    a. Pupillary size and reactivity
    b. Arousability
    c. Motor strength
    d. Posturing

Continued

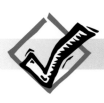

Makin' Money—Med-Surg Style
Questions—cont'd

MODERATE—cont'd

14. Which of the following is *not* a usual cause of seizures?
    a. Ingestion of toxins
    b. Acute MI
    c. Head trauma
    d. Alcohol withdrawal

15. Nonhemorrhagic stroke accounts for what percentage of all the strokes that occur?
    a. 80%
    b. 90%
    c. 50%
    d. 75%

16. Which of the following medications is indicated for seizure management?
    a. Zantac
    b. Lopressor
    c. Phenobarbital
    d. Fentanyl

17. The incident of stroke or brain attack causing death is which of the following?
    a. First leading cause of death
    b. Second leading cause of death
    c. Third leading cause of death
    d. Fourth leading cause of death

18. For embolic stroke, TPA (tissue plasminogen activator) must be administered within how many hours of symptom onset?
    a. 4 hours
    b. 1 hour
    c. 3 hours
    d. 5 hours

19. Which of the following is *not* typically present in the patient with acute stroke?
    a. Vertigo
    b. Anorexia
    c. Numbness of face, arm, or leg
    d. Seizures

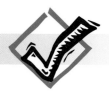

20. Pronator drift represents which of the following in the stroke patient?
    a. When the patient smiles or grimaces, the face droops on one side.
    b. When the patient closes the eyes with arms extended, downward movement of arm is present.
    c. Patient pulls your arm toward them and then pushes away. Weakness is present.
    d. The patient loses his or her underwear when they are lying prone.
21. Which of the following is a common cause of GI bleeding?
    a. Angina pectoris
    b. Pulmonary emboli
    c. Seizures
    d. Gastritis

DIFFICULT

1. Why are assessments of orthostatic vital signs important in the patient with a GI bleed?
    a. To assess patient LOC
    b. To estimate degree of acute blood loss
    c. To assess patient motor ability
    d. Because the doctor says so, that's why
2. Chest pain related to pulmonary embolus is most often the result of which of the following?
    a. Clots traveling from the lung to the heart
    b. Inflammation of the lining of the lungs
    c. Healing process after lung tissue is damaged
    d. Patient's fear of having to be poked with needles
3. Paradoxical chest movements indicate which of the following in a patient in trauma?
    a. Liver perforation
    b. Lung puncture
    c. Hemothorax
    d. Flail chest
4. Which of the following is an indicator of enlarging of an abdominal aortic aneurysm?
    a. Localized headache
    b. Absence of low back pain
    c. Inspiratory chest pain
    d. Abdominal pain radiating to neck

Continued

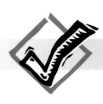

Makin' Money—Med-Surg Style Questions—cont'd

DIFFICULT—cont'd

5. Which of the following is administered to the patient with prolonged clotting times?
   a. Heparin
   b. Coumadin
   c. Vitamin K
   d. Lovenox

6. Patients with acute GI bleeds who require invasive procedures have which of the following mortality rates compared with the normal population?
   a. The same as the normal population
   b. Decreased
   c. Increased
   d. About 50% less than the normal population

7. Which is *not* an example of a space-occupying lesion of the brain?
   a. Tumor
   b. Embolic stroke
   c. Subdural hematoma
   d. Ruptured cerebral hematoma

8. The physiology of consciousness is controlled by what part of the brain?
   a. Cerebellum
   b. Cerebrum
   c. Hypothalamus
   d. Brain stem

9. Which of the following drugs can affect papillary reaction?
   a. Phenergan
   b. Morphine
   c. IV Lopressor
   d. Versed

10. Abnormal motor responses result from disruption of the corticospinal pathway from the cortex to what structure in the brain?
    a. Cerebellum
    b. Brain stem
    c. Hypothalamus
    d. Cerebrum

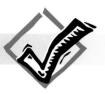

11. Which of the following is characteristic of a tonic-clonic seizure?
    a. Gradual onset
    b. Characterized by nonpurposeful movements of the extremities
    c. Does not result in loss of consciousness
    d. No memory loss usually seen after the seizure
12. Why are patients with acute stroke ordered to take nothing by mouth (NPO)?
    a. Allows for better assessment of LOC
    b. Decreases risk of aspiration
    c. Physician may need to draw fasting laboratory work
    d. It takes too much time to feed a stroke patient
13. Which of the following is *not* a complication of GI bleeding?
    a. Septic shock
    b. Anemia
    c. Hypovolemic shock
    d. Exsanguination
14. A blood loss of 1500 ml indicates what percentage of blood volume lost?
    a. Less than 10%
    b. 20% to 40%
    c. 50% to 60%
    d. 60% to 75%
15. A positive finding for orthostatic vital signs is what amount of change in the systolic BP reading?
    a. 8 mm Hg
    b. 5 mm Hg
    c. 10 mm Hg
    d. 20 mm Hg
16. What is the name of the syndrome in which severe retching is noted before onset of bleeding?
    a. Osler-Weber-Rendu disease
    b. Mallory-Weiss syndrome
    c. Dysphagia
    d. Abdominal aortic aneurism (AAA)
17. Blood loss of 1500 ml indicates which level of shock?
    a. Severe
    b. Moderate
    c. Mild
    d. No shock present

Continued

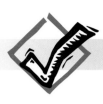

Makin' Money—Med-Surg Style Questions—cont'd

DIFFICULT—cont'd

18. What two abnormal laboratory values are commonly seen with the administration of stored blood?
    a. High potassium/high calcium
    b. High potassium/low calcium
    c. Low potassium/low calcium
    d. None of the above

19. Which of the following does *not* help determine the status of a patient with GI bleeding?
    a. Adequate tissue perfusion
    b. Urine output of at least 30 cc/hr
    c. Able to tolerate fluids
    d. Maintains a mean arterial pressure of 60 mm Hg

20. Which of the following is a complication of abdominal trauma?
    a. Septic shock
    b. Cardiogenic shock
    c. Hypovolemic shock
    d. Anaphylactic shock

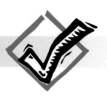

Makin' Money—Med-Surg Style Questions
ANSWERS

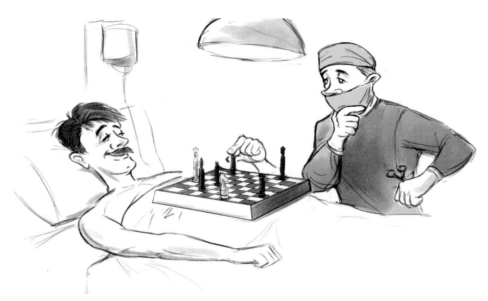

EASY

1. What can cause a change in papillary responsiveness?
   d. Brain stem lesions
2. Of the following, which situation would be least serious in the assessment of arousability?
   c. Arouses to name
3. In what situation would physician notification *not* be an immediate priority?
   a. Changes in vital signs
4. Which of the following best describes the type of pedal pulses seen in a patient with a dissecting abdominal aortic aneurysm?
   d. Absent
5. A sudden fullness in the throat followed by a rush of blood indicates which of the following?
   d. Esophageal varices
6. The color of stools in the patient with a lower GI bleed would be which of the following?
   c. Tarry
7. Which of the following is the location of the origin of the coronary arteries?
   d. Base of the aorta

Continued

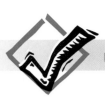

Makin' Money—Med-Surg Style Questions
ANSWERS—cont'd

EASY—cont'd

8. Shock is commonly associated in the patient with a systolic blood pressure of:
   b. 80 mm Hg
9. How does morphine relieve chest pain in the patient with an acute MI?
   a. Widens the diameter of the arteries of the heart
10. Which of the following is a common indicator of an abdominal aortic aneurysm?
    c. Pulsatile abdominal mass
11. The normal capillary refill is how many seconds?
    c. Less than 2
12. While replacing lost fluids, which of the following indicates fluid overload?
    b. CHF
13. The rhythm disturbance seen in acute MI that accounts for sudden death is which of the following?
    c. Ventricular fibrillation
14. Angina pectoris typically radiates to which of the following?
    b. Neck and jaw
15. How much urine does a typical adult produce per hour?
    b. 30 cc
16. Angina pain typically lasts how long?
    d. Less than 5 minutes
17. What does *exsanguination* mean?
    c. Rapid blood loss
18. How long do you wait between position changes when assessing orthostatic vital signs?
    c. 1 minute

MODERATE

1. Muffled or distant breath sounds can indicate which of the following?
   b. Hemothorax
2. The patient experiencing angina usually describes the pain as:
   a. Mild-to-moderate

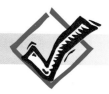

3. Which of the following is *not* a potential cause of a change in a patient's level of consciousness?
   d. Mild-to-moderate hypoglycemia

4. Which patient position is useful for the patient with a pulmonary embolus?
   c. Semi-Fowler's

5. In assessing a patient with an acute stroke, which of the following would *not* be your first priority?
   d. Assessment of vital signs

6. Which of the following would *not* result in papillary size and reaction?
   d. Pulmonary embolus

7. Which of the following can indicate fluid around the heart or pericardial tamponade?
   b. Muffled heart sounds

8. Which of the following indicates a positive finding for orthostatic systolic blood pressure changes?
   d. Decrease of 10 mm Hg

9. An appropriate definition of hemiparesis is which of the following?
   c. Weakness

10. Of the following, which is an early indicator of neurologic damage?
    c. Changes in LOC

11. Which of the following is *false* about status epilepticus?
    c. Usually does not require medication

12. What percentage of emboli develop from a blood clot?
    a. 99%

13. The assessment that indicates evaluation of level of consciousness is:
    b. Arousability

14. Which of the following is *not* a usual cause of seizures?
    b. Acute MI

15. Nonhemorrhagic stroke accounts for what percentage of all the strokes that occur?
    a. 80%

16. Which of the following medications is indicated for seizure management?
    c. Phenobarbital

17. The incident of stroke or brain attack causing death is which of the following?
    c. Third leading cause of death

Continued

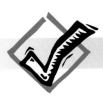

Makin' Money—Med-Surg Style Questions
ANSWERS—cont'd

MODERATE—cont'd

18. For embolic stroke, TPA must be administered within how many hours of symptom onset?
    c. 3 hours
19. Which of the following is *not* typically present in the patient with acute stroke?
    b. Anorexia
20. Pronator drift represents which of the following in the stroke patient?
    b. When the patient closes the eyes with arms extended, downward movement of arm is present.
21. Which of the following is a common cause of GI bleeding?
    d. Gastritis

DIFFICULT

1. Why are assessments of orthostatic vital signs important in the patient with a GI bleed?
   b. To estimate degree of acute blood loss
2. Chest pain related to pulmonary embolus is most often the result of which of the following?
   b. Inflammation of the lining of the lungs
3. Paradoxical chest movements indicate which of the following in a patient in trauma?
   d. Flail chest
4. Which of the following is an indicator of enlarging of an abdominal aortic aneurysm?
   d. Abdominal pain radiating to neck
5. Which of the following is administered to the patient with prolonged clotting times?
   c. Vitamin K
6. Patients with acute GI bleeds who require invasive procedures have which of the following mortality rates compared with the normal population?
   c. Increased
7. Which is *not* an example of a space-occupying lesion of the brain?
   b. Embolic stroke

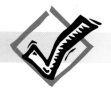

8. The physiology of consciousness is controlled by what part of the brain?
   b. Cerebrum
9. Which of the following drugs can affect papillary reaction?
   b. Morphine
10. Abnormal motor responses result from disruption of the cortico-spinal pathway from the cortex to what structure in the brain?
    b. Brain stem
11. Which of the following is characteristic of a tonic-clonic seizure?
    b. Characterized by nonpurposeful movements of the extremities
12. Why are patients with acute stroke kept NPO?
    b. Decreases risk of aspiration
13. Which of the following is *not* a complication of GI bleeding?
    a. Septic shock
14. A blood loss of 1500 ml indicates what percentage of blood volume lost?
    b. 20% to 40%
15. A positive finding for orthostatic vital signs is what amount of change in the systolic BP reading?
    c. 10 mm Hg
16. What is the name of the syndrome in which severe retching is noted before onset of bleeding?
    b. Mallory-Weiss syndrome
17. Blood loss of 1500 ml indicates which level of shock?
    b. Moderate
18. What two abnormal laboratory values are commonly seen with the administration of stored blood?
    b. High potassium/low calcium
19. Which of the following does *not* help determine the status of a patient with GI bleeding?
    c. Able to tolerate fluids
20. Which of the following is a complication of abdominal trauma?
    c. Hypovolemic shock

Fightin' Friends

15 to 30 minutes   Iris Trahan, RN, BSN, CCRN

Tool box
- **Two desk bells from an office supply store**
- **Flipchart for score keeping**
- **Two tables and chairs in the front of the room**
- **Fightin' Friends ready-to-use sheet and answer key**
- **Small prizes**

Educator secrets
Participants can be very competitive. It is helpful to have a panel of judges to help validate whether specific answers are acceptable or to decide which team member rang in first. The panel should be experts in the field related to course content.

Preparation

1. Write questions about the content you want to review. Include multiple-answer and single-answer questions.
2. Set up the table or cart in the front of the room.
3. Place one of the bells on each table.

Implementation

1. Choose two teams, each with four to six members. Initially ask for volunteers or copy the sign-in sheet and randomly draw names for each team.
2. Ask each team to come up with a creative name such as The V Tachs versus the GI Bleeds.
3. Position team members at opposing tables in the front of the room facing each other.
4. Each team member takes a turn coming up to the table to possibly answer the questions by ringing in first.
5. The coordinator reads the question. (Example: The coordinator reads a scenario with a patient who has decreased hematocrit and hemoglobin (H&H) and bloody diarrhea. Diagnosis of a GI bleed is correct.) If the first person to ring in answers the question correctly, his or her team has the opportunity to answer subsequent questions to gain more points for that round. Each question has a point value, with more difficult questions being worth more points.
6. The team is asked the multiple-answer question. (Example: Name four other signs and symptoms commonly seen with an acute GI bleed.) Each team member is called upon one at a time to give one answer. If a team member is unable to give the correct answer, the team receives one "punch" against their team. After three punches, the opposing team can try to give the right answer and steal all the points won by their opposition thus far.
7. Play continues until time is up. The winner of the game is the team with the most points. Prizes can be given to all, or specific prizes can be given to winners and to second-place team.

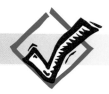

Fightin' Friends Questions

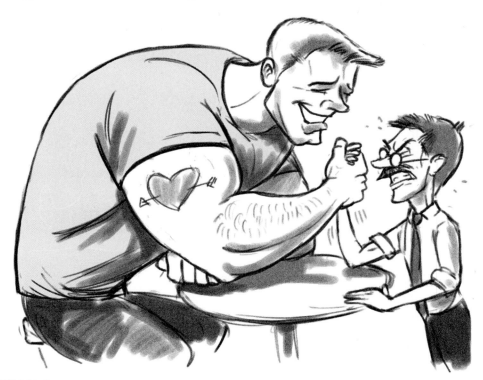

DIRECTIONS: Select the correct answer for each question (some questions have more than one correct answer). Give yourself 5 points for EACH correct answer.

Questions	Points Earned
1. What is the typical statement used by a patient to describe the chest heaviness related to the heart?	_____
2. Name seven things that tend to cause angina pectoris.	_____
3. How is the severity of chest pain by the patient who is experiencing angina typically described?	_____
4. What are three things that occur in the coronary artery for an acute MI to occur?	_____
5. What period of time does the pain of angina pectoris last?	_____
6. Other than chest pain, what are four other signs or symptoms of an acute MI?	_____

Continued

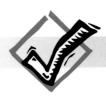

Fightin' Friends Questions—cont'd

Questions   **Points Earned**

7. What two things typically relieve angina pain?   _____

8. Identify five sites to which angina pectoris pain can radiate.   _____

9. How long does the pain of an acute MI typically last?   _____

10. Describe two reasons why an acute MI can cause pulmonary edema.   _____

11. Why is the sputum bloody in acute pulmonary edema?   _____

Two-Part Question

12. a. Name two causes of pulmonary edema other than the heart.   _____

    b. Describe the two ways it causes pulmonary edema.   _____

13. The systolic blood pressure in shock is typically what reading?   _____

14. Identify eight signs and symptoms of pulmonary edema. *(40 possible total points)*   _____

15. What is the most common cause of death after an acute MI?   _____

16. Identify two priorities of care for the patient with angina pectoris.   _____

17. What do the letters *PTCA* stand for?   _____

18. Identify two priorities of care for the patient with acute MI.   _____

19. What is another name for coronary artery disease (CAD)? *(Learner must spell it out to be correct.)*   _____

20. What two things does nitroglycerin do that helps the heart?   _____

21. Where do the coronary arteries originate?   _____

22. What do the letters *P-Q-R-S-T* stand for in pain assessment? *(All must be correct to count as correct.)*   _____

23. What is another word for lack of oxygen in the heart?   _____

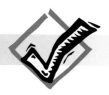

Questions   **Points Earned**

24. Name the six key points that should be   _____
    considered when nitroglycerin is
    administered. *(30 points total)*
25. What two positions are most effective in   _____
    helping the breathing of a patient with
    acute pulmonary edema?
26. What do the letters *M-O-N-A* in the acute MI   _____
    treatment stand for?
27. Why do the two positions named in   _____
    question 25 help the patient? *(15 points total)*
28. What are two priorities of care for the patient   _____
    in pulmonary edema?
29. Which of the following represents the   _____
    mortality from acute pulmonary embolus?
    a. 75% to 80%
    b. 50% to 75%
    c. 30% to 35%
    d. 90% to 95%
30. Name seven other sources of emboli other   _____
    than a blood clot.
31. What percentage of emboli develop from a   _____
    blood clot?
    a. 75%
    b. 99%
    c. 70%
    d. 90%
32. Identify risk factors for pulmonary embolus.   _____
33. Anticoagulants do what two things in the   _____
    setting of pulmonary embolus?
34. What four characteristics of pain are the   _____
    result of pulmonary embolus?
35. What two diagnostic studies are used in the   _____
    diagnosis of acute pulmonary embolism
    and where they are done? *(Both must be
    named to earn points.)*
36. Name seven symptoms of pulmonary   _____
    embolus other than those discussed
    previously.

Continued

185

Fightin' Friends Questions—cont'd

Questions   **Points Earned**

Bonus question: 10 Points (for the team in second place)

37. On weekends and holidays, who has the   _____
    authority to authorize calling in the on-call
    team members?

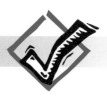

Fightin' Friends Questions
ANSWER KEY

1. What is the typical statement used by a patient to describe the chest heaviness related to the heart?
   "It feels like an elephant is sitting on my chest."
2. Name seven things that tend to cause angina pectoris.
   (1) Exertion
   (2) Anxiety
   (3) Cold weather
   (4) Blood loss
   (5) Heavy meal
   (6) Carbon monoxide
   (7) Trauma
3. How is the severity of chest pain by the patient who is experiencing angina typically described?
   Mild to moderate
4. What are three things that occur in the coronary artery for an acute MI to occur?
   (1) Plaque rupture
   (2) Exposure of the artery lumen to platelets
   (3) Development of a blood clot at the site
5. What period of time does the pain of angina pectoris last?
   Less than 5 minutes
6. Other than chest pain, what are four other signs or symptoms of an acute MI?
   (1) Diaphoresis
   (2) Shortness of breath
   (3) GI upset
   (4) Feeling of impending doom
7. What two things typically relieve angina pain?
   (1) Rest
   (2) Nitroglycerine
8. Identify five sites to which angina pectoris pain can radiate.
   (1) Left arm
   (2) Jaw
   (3) Neck
   (4) Shoulder
   (5) Epigastrium
9. How long does the pain of an acute MI typically last?
   Longer than 5 minutes

Continued

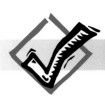

Fightin' Friends Questions
ANSWER KEY—cont'd

10. Describe two reasons why an acute MI can cause pulmonary edema.
   (1) Inadequate pump
   (2) Fluid overload
11. Why is the sputum bloody in acute pulmonary edema?
   The increased pressure in the lungs causes blood vessels in the lungs to rupture.

Two-Part Question

12. a. Name two causes of pulmonary edema other than the heart.
      (1) Increased salt intake
      (2) Impaired renal function
    b. Describe the two ways it causes pulmonary edema.
      (1) Causes fluid retention that strains the heart
      (2) Fluid overload results from kidneys' failure to remove fluid from the bloodstream
13. The systolic blood pressure in shock is typically what reading?
   Less than 80 mm Hg
14. Identify eight signs and symptoms of pulmonary edema.
   (1) SOB while lying flat
   (2) Respiratory distress
   (3) Weakness
   (4) Cool, clammy skin
   (5) Decreased LOC
   (6) Frothy, bloody sputum
   (7) Rapid irregular pulse
   (8) Wheezes and crackles in the lungs
15. What is the most common cause of death after an acute MI?
   Ventricular fibrillation
16. Identify two priorities of care for the patient with angina pectoris.
   (1) Relief of the acute angina attack
   (2) Reduce the risk of an acute MI
17. What do the letters PTCA stand for?
   Percutaneous transluminal coronary angioplasty
18. Identify two priorities of care for the patient with acute MI.
   (1) Increase blood flow to the heart
   (2) Increase the oxygen concentration of the blood
19. What is another name for coronary artery disease (CAD)?
   Atherosclerosis

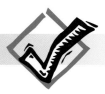

20. What two things does nitroglycerin do that helps the heart?
    (1) Dilates or widens the blood vessels
    (2) Increases blood flow to the heart
21. Where do the coronary arteries originate?
    At the base of the aorta
22. What do the letters *P-Q-R-S-T* stand for in pain assessment?
    P—provocation
    Q—quality
    R—radiation
    S—severity
    T—timing
23. What is another word for lack of oxygen in the heart?
    Ischemia
24. Name the six key points that should be considered when nitro-glycerin is administered.
    (1) One tablet under tongue
    (2) Given at 3-minute intervals
    (3) Make patient lie down before administration
    (4) Must burn under the tongue to be considered good
    (5) Total of three tablets every 5 minutes
    (6) If no relief with three tablets, immediately go to the emergency department
25. What two positions are most effective in helping the breathing of a patient with acute pulmonary edema?
    (1) Elevate the head of the bed
    (2) Dangle the legs over the side of the bed
26. What do the letters *M-O-N-A* in the acute MI treatment stand for?
    M—morphine
    O—oxygen
    N—nitroglycerin
    A—aspirin
27. Why do the two positions named in question 25 help the patient?
    (1) Increases lung capacity and ease of breathing
    (2) Pools blood in the patient's extremities
28. What are two priorities of care for the patient in pulmonary edema?
    (1) Decrease blood volume returning to the heart
    (2) Improve pumping ability of the heart

Continued

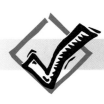

Fightin' Friends Questions
ANSWER KEY—cont'd

29. Which of the following represents the mortality from acute pulmonary embolus?
    c. 30% to 35%
30. Name seven other sources of emboli other than a blood clot.
    (1) Tumors
    (2) Air
    (3) Fat
    (4) Bone marrow
    (5) Amniotic fluid
    (6) Septic emboli
    (7) Vegetation on heart valves
31. What percentage of emboli develop from a blood clot?
    b. 99%
32. Identify risk factors for pulmonary embolus.?
    (1) Pelvic or leg surgery
    (2) Pelvic or leg trauma
    (3) Deep vein thrombosis (DVT) or a history of DVT
    (4) Obesity
    (5) Estrogen therapy
    (6) Clotting abnormalities
    (7) Cancer (malignancy)
33. Anticoagulants do what two things in the setting of pulmonary embolus?
    (1) Decrease incidence of future clots
    (2) Slow the development of thrombi onto emboli
34. What four characteristics of pain are the result of pulmonary embolus?
    (1) Sudden onset
    (2) Related to breathing
    (3) Worse with deep breath/inspiration
    (4) Not improved by positioning
35. What two diagnostic studies are used in the diagnosis of acute pulmonary embolism, and where are the studies done?
    (1) Lung scan: Nuclear medicine
    (2) Pulmonary angiogram: Special procedures in radiology or catheterization laboratory

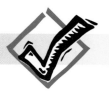

36. Name seven symptoms of pulmonary embolus other than those discussed previously.
    (1) Increased respiratory rate
    (2) Increased heart rate
    (3) Syncope
    (4) Apprehension
    (5) Hemoptysis
    (6) Dyspnea
    (7) Feeling of impending doom
37. On weekends and holidays, who has the authority to authorize calling in the on-call team members?
    The house supervisor or administrative representative on call for the house is authorized.

Elements of Protocol Crossword Puzzle

Jeri Ashley, RN, MSN, AOCN, CCRC

10 to 15 minutes

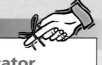

Tool box
- **Elements of Protocol Crossword Puzzle**
- **One pen or pencil per learner**
- **Answer key**

Preparation

1. Make a copy of the ready-to-use Elements of Protocol Crossword Puzzle for each participant.
2. Use this as an introduction to the lesson, a review after the lesson, or as part of your required annual training.
3. Make sure all participants have a pen or pencil.
4. Make a copy of the answer key.

Implementation

1. Distribute the crossword puzzle.
2. Challenge your learners to complete the puzzle as individuals or as teams.
3. If energy and attention are low during your lesson presentation, stop and let your participants engage in this energizing activity.
4. Crossword puzzles can act as pre- or posttests, and they can also be sent out days or weeks after the lesson as reinforcement of important concepts.

Variation

1. Use a poster printer copy machine to turn the crossword into a poster-sized image.
2. Plan for groups of two to six to discuss and fill in a poster-sized copy of the crossword puzzle before or after your lesson.

Educator secrets
If you have different ability levels in your session, pair learners to maximize benefits to all participants.

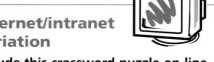

Internet/intranet variation

Include this crossword puzzle on-line in a course as a pretest or posttest.

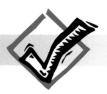

Elements of Protocol Crossword Puzzle

DIRECTIONS: Complete the crossword puzzle using the clues provided on pages 194 and 195.

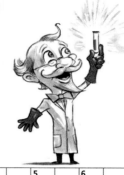

Continued

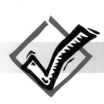

Elements of Protocol Crossword Puzzle—cont'd

Across

2. This section of a protocol provides a description of the prospective monitoring system built into the study. This monitoring system is designed to assess the completeness and accuracy of everything in the study, such as eligibility criteria, and reporting deadlines for serious adverse events.

7. According to www.webster.com, "The power to produce an effect." In a protocol, examining diagnostic results, survival, and clinical responses does the assessment of this criterion. Additionally, the timing or schedule for these assessments is also included here.

9. The principles of conduct guiding the investigators, clinical research coordinators, sponsors, and others in the performance of the clinical trial. Specific issues that may be addressed in this section includes dose modifications, compliance issues, patients lost to follow-up, early discontinuation of the trial, medical emergencies, and confidentiality of data.

13. These documents are original documents, data, or records in which subject information is initially recorded—either written or electronically.

14. This describes the methodology used to achieve goals and objectives of the clinical trials. This element of a protocol included the study endpoints, study schema, the study procedures, and the steps outlined for completing the study.

15. An outcome measurement used frequently in oncology clinical trials; may be defined as a time interval between start of study drug to death.

16. These elements in a protocol can be primary, secondary, or exploratory, and they define the purpose or focus of the trial.

17. Organizing a trial plan so that it includes multiple clinical centers participating in the research study. This is useful in replicating clinical practice across a country or countries.

18. A noun meaning written evidence kept in a record that can be used to prove or support an event or an agreement.

20. This is a description of the experimental intervention under study; it will include the drugs, dose, route of administration, schedule of administration, toxicities, medications that need to be used in addition to study drug, and procedures to monitor for compliance.

22. The assignment of patients to treatment interventions in a random manner, "like the flip of a coin." Also called *random assignment.*

24. The rate at which patients are enrolled into a particular clinical trial as measured in a specified period of time such as a month.

25. This element of a protocol contains a description of external funding for a protocol; could also include plans by the sponsor to pay stipends to patients or institutions. In most cases, this is kept as a separate document from the clinical proposal.

26. This part of a protocol describes the statistical and administrative procedures for monitoring the progress of a trial to implement early termination.

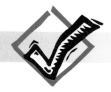

27. This describes what documents and data are maintained and by whom; this could refer to handling of data or regulatory management.
28. A noun describing the action a sponsor or investigator may take to remove a patient from study; the patient may also do this and terminate his or her involvement in a clinical trial.

Down

1. This section of a protocol contains information found on the face sheet plus one to two pages that follow. The information found there includes the protocol identification number and contact information for key individuals, agencies, sponsor, and monitors.
3. A noun describing a sum paid out as compensation for damage, injury, or loss; this is a protocol element that is defined in the financial contract.
4. The abbreviation for clinical research coordinator.
5. Often referred to as the "n," this describes the amount of enrollees involved in a clinical trial and is a statistical element of a protocol. It is also referred to as the sample size.
6. A noun meaning to fall back or sink again; in cancer terminology, it describes a return of cancer after a remission or a worsening of the disease.

8. A noun defining a course or principle of action adopted or proposed by a government, party, business, or individual. In the case of a protocol, this defined course of action usually refers to what, when, and how an investigator may publish information about a study or the study drug.
10. This section of a protocol specifies the parameters to be taken to prevent injuries to a subject; it will include methods and timing for assessments and also the post-treatment follow-up schedule.
11. Subdividing a population of subjects according to some characteristic such as sex, age group, or previous treatment or treatments for the disease being studied.
12. The estimated length of a clinical trial in terms of time.
18. Abbreviation for data manager.
19. Additional information or documents. This could include the informed consent form, documents addressing multi-center logistics issues, or any appendices.
21. These are outcomes that will be measured in a clinical trial and could include response to therapy, disease-free survival, or overall survival. The clinical and biologic parameters that are measured to evaluate the study's objectives.
23. The objective of a clinical trial; the aim of the protocol.

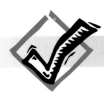

Elements of Protocol Crossword Puzzle
ANSWER KEY

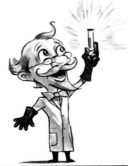

G									Q	U	A	L	I	T	Y	C	O	N	T	R	O	L			
E	F	F	I	C	A	C	Y							N			R		U		E				P
N														S			C		M		L				O
E	T	H	I	C	S							S		U					B		A				L
R					A							T		R					E		P				I
A					F							R		A		D			R		S	O	U	R	C	E
L				D	E	S	I	G	N			A		N		U			O		E				Y
I					T							T		C		R			F					
N					Y							I		E		A			S					
F												F				T		S	U	R	V	I	V	A	L
O	B	J	E	C	T	I	V	E	S			I				I			B					
R												E				O			J					
M	U	L	T	I	C	E	N	T	E	R	D	E	S	I	G	N			E					
A															D	O	C	U	M	E	N	T	S	
T	R	E	A	T	M	E	N	T	P	L	A	N				M		T					U
I			N															S					P
O		R	A	N	D	O	M	I	Z	A	T	I	O	N									P
N			D																				L
	P		O							A	C	C	R	U	A	L	R	A	T	E			E
	U		F	I	N	A	N	C	I	N	G												M
	R		N																				E
	P		T																				N
	O		S	T	O	P	P	I	N	G	R	U	L	E	S								T
	S																						S
R	E	C	O	R	D	K	E	E	P	I	N	G			W	I	T	H	D	R	A	W	A	L

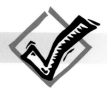

Across

2. Quality control
7. Efficacy
9. Ethics
13. Source
14. Design
15. Survival
16. Objectives
17. Multicenter design
18. Documents
20. Treatment plan
22. Randomization
24. Accrual rate
25. Financing
26. Stopping rules
27. Recordkeeping
28. Withdrawal

Down

1. General information
3. Insurance
4. CRC
5. Number of subjects
6. Relapse
8. Policy
10. Safety
11. Stratified
12. Duration
18. DM
19. Supplements
21. Endpoints
23. Purpose

TOPIC: Death and loss

The Death Exercise

Jeri L. Ashley, RN, MSN, AOCN, CCRC

20 to 30 minutes

Tool box
- **The Death Exercise Script with questions**
- **Watch with second hand or timing device**

Preparation

1. This exercise can be used in a variety of settings for a variety of reasons. It can be used to assist others in understanding the loss experienced in illness, to stress the importance of family and significant others, and to aid in bringing death to one's conscious mind as a reality.
2. Copy the Death Exercise Script with questions.
3. Ready the timing device.

Implementation

1. Read the script quietly without a great deal of inflection and fluctuation in the voice. This will not distract the participants with changes in the reader's voice.
2. Read the script and use the timing device to stop for the recommended times listed on the script.
3. At the end, foster a discussion with the group using the questions that follow the script.
4. Be available after the activity to talk to participants one on one.

Educator secrets
This is a powerful and emotional activity for those who experience it. Be ready for a variety of experiences.

Internet/intranet variation
This can be posted with the questions in an Internet/Intranet course.

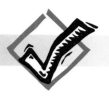

The Death Exercise Script

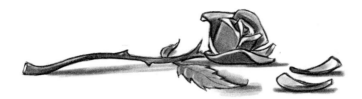

"I am now going to provide you with an opportunity to enter into an imagery experience that will allow you to gain a few insights into the lives of your patients (clients, family members, church members, and so on)."

"If you choose not to participate, please sit quietly so that you will not distract others around you who do want to do this exercise."

"First, please get into a comfortable position that will enable you to relax." (If appropriate and available, encourage participants to use the floor, chairs, tables, or couches to become physically comfortable.)

"When you become comfortable, please relax and close your eyes. Take several deep breaths and release the air slowly." (Wait a few seconds while participants relax.)

"I am going to request that you pay close attention only to the sound of my voice and the words that I am saying to you. Should you become distracted by other sounds in the room, acknowledge them and then return your attention to my voice." (Wait a few seconds while participants note other sounds in the room.)

"Now imagine a hospital room. You are reclining in the hospital bed. You are the patient. For the purpose of this imaginary experience, please choose a chronic, terminal illness." (Wait a few seconds while participants choose their illness.)

"Your physician has just entered your room and explained to you that you have a very serious illness and that you have only 1 year to live." (Allow a period of time to pass that is 1 minute or less—usually 15 to 30 seconds is sufficient.)

"Some time has passed, and now you have only 9 months to live." (Wait 1 minute or less—usually 15 to 30 seconds is sufficient.)

Continued

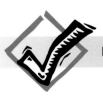

The Death Exercise Script—cont'd

"Some more time has passed, and now you have only 6 months to live. Note your location. Are you at home, at the hospital, or in a nursing home?" (Wait 1 minute or less—usually 15 to 30 seconds is sufficient.)

"More time has passed, and now you have 3 months to live. Note that you are losing some physical capabilities and that your physical appearance has changed: you have lost weight, you are pale, and you feel tired all of the time." (Wait 1 minute or less—usually 15 to 30 seconds is sufficient.)

"You now have 1 month to live. Again, note where you are. You are now having some physical symptoms such as pain, nausea and vomiting, weakness and fatigue. Who is with you?" (Wait 1 minute or less—usually 15 to 30 seconds is sufficient.)

"You now have 1 week to live. Where are you and who is with you?" (Wait 1 minute or less—usually 15 to 30 seconds is sufficient.)

"You now have 3 days to live. Who is with you?" (Wait 1 minute or less—usually 15 to 30 seconds is sufficient.)

"You have 1 day to live." (Wait 1 minute.)

"You may now open your eyes." (Give the participants a few seconds to "come back" into the room.)

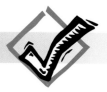

Discussion Questions

1. Where were you throughout the experience?
2. Who was with you in the hospital room when the physician gave you the news?
3. Was there anyone who was consistently with you throughout the experience?
4. Who was with you at the end?
5. What was the last day like?
6. Are there any particular feelings that you had throughout the experience?
7. Is there anything else that you would like to share with us?

"I am going to ask that if you need to discuss this experience further, I will be around after this session to hear your story." (This activity can be an emotional one, and offering this opportunity for them to "talk it out" creates an environment for them to process what they just experienced.)

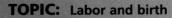

Labor is Like a Bouncing Ball

10 to 20 minutes

Cecelia Deslauriers, RN, CLC, IBCLC, BS

Tool box

- **One brown paper bag and paper clip per class participant (plus one for the educator)**
- **A variety of balls: ball with superhero inside, ball with angles, ball with suction cups, neon-colored ping-pong ball, golf ball, ball that looks like a rock, koosh ball, ball filled with liquid, hackey sack ball, ball with smiley face, ball with sad face and closed eyes, earth ball, ball with a fish on it, bag with two or three balls in it, inflatable ball, ball with a "C" on it, and any other ball that has an association with childbirth.**

Preparation

1. Place a ball in each bag, and seal the end of the bag with a paper clip. To represent twins or triplets, place two or three balls in one of the bags.
2. Randomly place the brown paper bags on the floor in the middle of the room, making sure there are enough bags for everyone in your group to choose one (including you, the educator).

Implementation

1. Make the analogy that all pregnant women look the same from the outside, just like the brown paper bags. The bags are closed with a paper clip to represent a closed cervix.
2. Ask both pregnant mothers and their support persons to randomly select a bag. You should also select a bag and participate.
3. Tell the group they are allowed to shake the bag but are not to feel the contents.
4. Ask each person (or a few volunteers) to guess the contents.
5. Explain that each person is to observe what happens when the contents of their bag is released.
6. At a given signal, invite everyone to open the bags, hold it above their heads, and drop the contents onto the floor at the same time.
7. Say, "Ready, set, drop!" Release the contents of your bag when everyone else does.
8. Comment on the ball from your bag with reference to the birthing process, and ask the participants to do the same.
9. Some examples and what each might represent:
   - Ball with superhero inside—A very powerful, challenging labor
   - Ball with angles—Rolls in unpredictable directions; different from what the doctor expected, with complications or other conditions arising

- Ball with suction cups—Will stick to a wall or a window and represents arrested labor
- Neon-colored ping pong ball—Bright, light, and quick to rebound in the early stages of labor
- Golf ball—Lots of dimples and a high bounce represents frequent bouts or prelabor contractions and then the real thing
- Rock ball—A road block that gives the mother time to reassess, or become easier
- Koosh ball—Drops and does not bounce (represents failure to progress)
- Liquid-filled ball—Rupture of membranes
- Square hackey sack ball—A labor that does not follow the pattern of normal labors
- Ball with a smiley face—Easy labor
- Ball with a sad face and closed eyes—Transition
- Earth ball—Reminder that women are giving birth all around the world (feel the fellowship of motherhood or parenthood)
- Ball with a fish on it—Water birth, water tub for labor, shower
- Bag with two or three balls in it—Twins or triplets or the difference between primips and multips labor
- Inflatable ball—The birthing ball for back labor
- Ball with a "C" on it—Cesarean birth

10. Use the learners' responses to provide a springboard for discussions and proactive problem solving.
11. Be aware they will identify their fears, past experiences, and hopes and realize they are not alone in their feelings. Some multips will share which ball represented their previous labors.

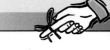

Educator secrets
This activity relaxes everyone and makes discussion of birth possibilities flow more easily.

PART 5
Instant Internet and Intranet Ideas

What is the Sequence Here?

Michele L. Deck, RN, MEd, BSN, LCCE, FACCE

1 to 2 minutes

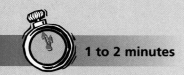

Tool box

- **What is the Sequence Here? ready-to-use sheet**
- **Written module or Internet/ intranet course**
- **What is the Sequence Here? Answer Key**

Preparation

1. Copy the What is the Sequence Here? ready-to-use sheet into the beginning of a written module or Internet/intranet course.
2. Copy the What is the Sequence Here? Answer Key into one of the last pages or screens of a written module or Internet/intranet course.
3. Reference the page number where the answer can be found on the What is the Sequence Here? ready-to-use sheet into the beginning of a written module or Internet/intranet course, so learners can check their answers.
4. Personalize the message at the end of the activity.
5. Continue with the information in the course or module.

Implementation

1. Distribute written modules or ready your on-line course.
2. Answer any questions that may arise from the activity.

Educator secrets

Thought-provoking activities such as these can warm up the thought process before the learners begin reading content information. You can also use this as a thought starter in a live class.

206

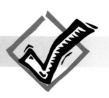

What Is the Sequence Here?

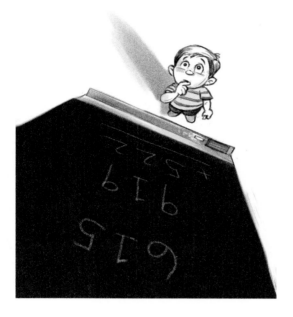

DIRECTIONS: The numbers 0 through 15 are in the following sequence. The missing numbers are 0, 7, and 9. Complete the following series of numbers by placing these missing numbers where they belong in the sequence:

8, 11, 15, 5, 4, 14, ___, 1, ___, 6, 10, 13, 3, 2, 12, ____

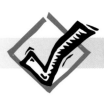

What Is the Sequence Here?
ANSWER KEY

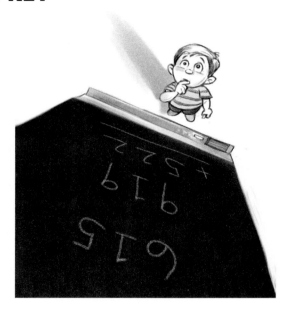

8, 11, 15, 5, 4, 14, <u>9</u>, 1, <u>7</u>, 6, 10, 13, 3, 2, 12, <u>0</u>

The sequence of the numbers is alphabetical:

Eight

Eleven

Fifteen

Five

Four

Fourteen

<u>Nine</u>

One

<u>Seven</u>

Six

Ten

Thirteen

Three

Two

Twelve

<u>Zero</u>

Sometimes it is easy to be confused by written information. This course will present a variety of important information to make you more effective in your job. Please read through the information carefully and pay attention to the small details. Enjoy the course!

Memorizing Code

Michele L. Deck, RN, MEd, BSN, LCCE, FACCE

1 to 2 minutes

Preparation

1. Copy the Memorizing Code ready-to-use sheet into the beginning of a written module or Internet/intranet course.
2. Copy the Memorizing Code Answer Key into one of the last pages or screens of a written module or Internet/intranet course.
3. Reference the page number where the answer can be found on the Memorizing Code ready-to-use sheet into the beginning of a written module or Internet/intranet course, so learners can check their answers.
4. Personalize the message at the end of the activity.
5. Continue with the information in the course or module.

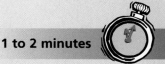

Tool box
- **Memorizing Code ready-to-use sheet**
- **Written module or Internet/intranet course**
- **Memorizing Code Answer Key**

Implementation

1. Distribute written modules or ready your on-line course.
2. Answer any questions that may arise from the activity.

Educator secrets
Thought-provoking activities such as these can warm up the thought process before the learners begin reading content information. You can also use this as a thought starter in a live class.

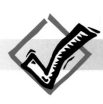

Memorizing Code

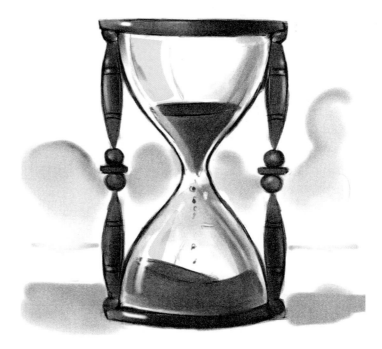

How long will it take you to memorize the following code, so you could use it without the following chart?

1 = ⌐

2 = ⊔

3 = ∟

4 = ⌐

5 = □

6 = [

7 = ⌐

8 = ⊓

9 = Γ

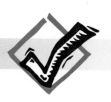

Memorizing Code
ANSWER KEY

If you were to draw a tic-tac-toe board as shown and were to list the numbers in sequence in it, you would have the key to the code. It is very easy to understand and it makes sense.

1	2	3
4	5	6
7	8	9

As you begin this course, you might be thinking it is hard to learn or that parts of the topic may not seem to make sense. However, just as the tic-tac-toe board looks difficult to learn in pieces, when it is all linked together it gives you an overall picture that makes sense. The same is true for this course. It will make sense and be easy to remember when you have the whole picture. Enjoy the course!

Recognizing Patterns

Michele L. Deck, RN, MEd, BSN, LCCE, FACCE

1 to 2 minutes

Preparation

1. Copy the Recognizing Patterns ready-to-use sheet into the beginning of a written module or Internet/intranet course.
2. Reference the page number where the answer can be found on the Recognizing Code ready-to-use sheet into the beginning of a written module or Internet/intranet course, so learners can check their answers.
3. Personalize the message at the end of the activity.
4. Continue with the information in the course or module.

Implementation

1. Distribute written modules or ready your on-line course.
2. Answer any questions that may arise from the activity.

Tool box
- Recognizing Patterns ready-to-use sheet
- Written module or Internet/intranet course
- Recognizing Patterns Answer Key

Educator secrets
Thought-provoking activities such as these can warm up the thought process before the learners begin reading content information. You can also use this as a thought starter in a live class.

212

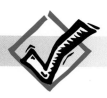

Recognizing Patterns

What do you see following?

- Boxes
- A train
- A bracelet
- What else?

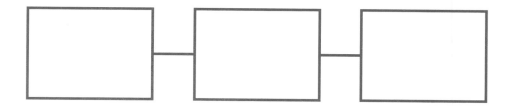

Do you see Hs now? Look at the highlighted areas:

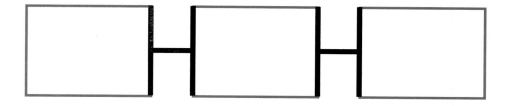

Look at this new figure. What do you see?

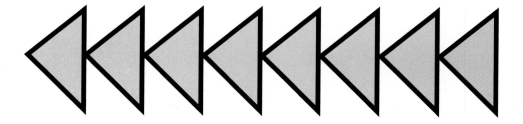

Do you at first see Ks?

Why is it possible to see many options in the top and middle illustrations, but you immediately see Ks in the bottom illustration? Is it possible that when you are made aware of a pattern, it makes it easier to see other patterns? This course will help you to recognize trends and patterns that were previously not perceived. Enjoy the course!

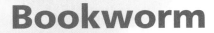

Bookworm

Michele L. Deck, RN, MEd, BSN, LCCE, FACCE

1 to 2 minutes

Tool box
- **Bookworm ready-to-use sheet**
- **Written module or Internet/intranet course**
- **Bookworm Answer Key**

Preparation

1. Copy the Bookworm ready-to-use sheet into the beginning of a written module or Internet/intranet course.
2. Copy the Bookworm Answer Key into one of the last pages or screens of a written module or Internet/intranet course.
3. Reference the page number where the answer can be found on the Bookworm ready-to-use sheet into the beginning of a written module or Internet/intranet course, so learners can check their answers.
4. Personalize the message at the end of the activity.
5. Continue with the information in the course or module.

Implementation

1. Distribute written modules or ready your on-line course.
2. Answer any questions that may arise from the activity.

Educator secrets
Thought-provoking activities such as these can warm up the thought process before the learners begin reading content information. You can also use this as a thought starter in a live class.

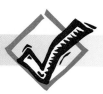

Bookworm

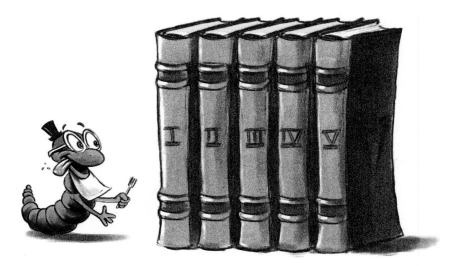

The previous figure shows five volumes of a policy and procedure manual sitting on a shelf in your facility. If the bookworm begins eating at page one of volume I and continues to eat through the last page of volume V, how many inches does the bookworm eat?

Each cover is $1/4$ inch thick.

From first page to last page, each volume is 2 inches thick.

How many inches does the bookworm eat?

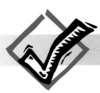
Bookworm
ANSWER KEY

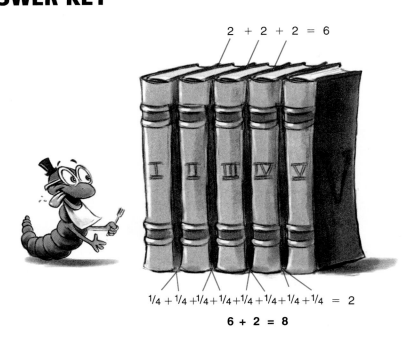

$$2 + 2 + 2 = 6$$

$$\tfrac{1}{4} + \tfrac{1}{4} + \tfrac{1}{4} + \tfrac{1}{4} + \tfrac{1}{4} + \tfrac{1}{4} + \tfrac{1}{4} + \tfrac{1}{4} = 2$$

6 + 2 = 8

Look at how the books are arranged on the shelf. The first page of Volume I is on the inside cover of the book. The last page of Volume V is on the inside cover. The correct answer is 8. Let's count:

Covers in inches:
- Volume I front cover—$\tfrac{1}{4}$ inch
- Volume II front cover—$\tfrac{1}{4}$ inch
- Pages, Volume II—2 inches
- Volume II back cover—$\tfrac{1}{4}$ inch
- Volume III front cover—$\tfrac{1}{4}$ inch
- Pages, Volume III—2 inches
- Volume III back cover— $\tfrac{1}{4}$ inch
- Volume IV front cover—$\tfrac{1}{4}$ inch
- Pages, Volume IV—2 inches
- Volume IV back cover—$\tfrac{1}{4}$ inch
- Volume V front cover—$\tfrac{1}{4}$ inch

The covers are $\tfrac{1}{4} + \tfrac{1}{4} + \tfrac{1}{4} + \tfrac{1}{4} + \tfrac{1}{4} + \tfrac{1}{4} + \tfrac{1}{4} + \tfrac{1}{4} = 2$

The pages are $2 + 2 + 2 = 6$

$2 + 6 = 8$

The answer is 8.

It is very important when measuring or calibrating that we begin at the correct point. This course will help you to learn the right starting point for your information and practice. Enjoy the course!

216

Housing Horses

Michele L. Deck, RN, MEd, BSN, LCCE, FACCE

Preparation

1. Copy the Housing Horses ready-to-use sheet into the beginning of a written module or Internet/intranet course.
2. Copy the Housing Horses Answer Key into one of the last pages or screens of a written module or Internet/intranet course.
3. Reference the page number where the answer can be found on the Housing Horses ready-to-use sheet into the beginning of a written module or Internet/intranet course, so learners can check their answers.
4. Personalize the message at the end of the activity.
5. Continue with the information in the course or module.

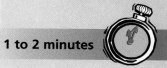

Tool box
- **Housing Horses ready-to-use sheet**
- **Written module or Internet/ intranet course**
- **Housing Horses Answer Key**

Implementation

1. Distribute written modules or ready your on-line course.
2. Answer any questions that may arise from the activity.

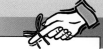

Educator secrets
Thought-provoking activities such as these can warm up the thought process before the learners begin reading content information. You can also use this as a thought starter in a live class.

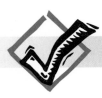

Housing Horses

You own 10 horses. Your stable has only nine stalls as seen following. Your job is to equally space the 10 horses in the nine stalls.

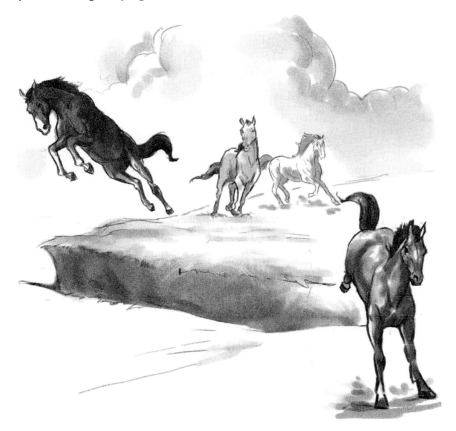

Here are the conditions:
- No two or more horses can be in the same stall at the same time.
- All horses must be housed simultaneously.
- No construction or destruction of the stalls is allowed.
- No killing of animals is allowed under any circumstances.

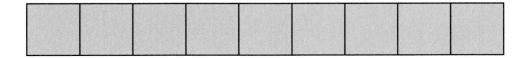

How can you equally space the 10 horses in the nine stalls?

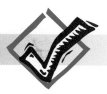

Housing Horses
ANSWER KEY

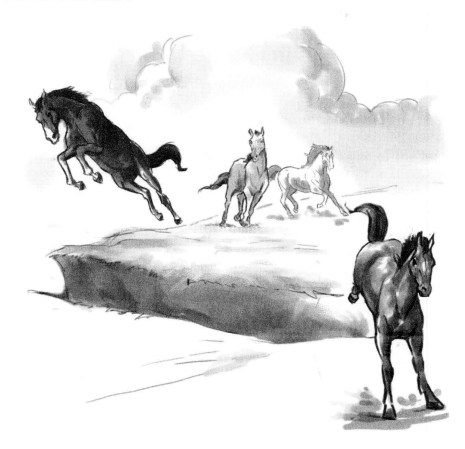

T	E	N	H	O	R	S	E	S

Are the 10 horses equally spaced in the nine stalls? Yes, they are, but many people are surprised by this solution.

To get this answer, you have to approach this problem from a different perspective. Sometimes we must approach a problem from a new angle or perspective to get an answer that works for a variety of people and situations. Take a new perspective on this course, and enjoy!

Month Math

Michele L. Deck, RN, MEd, BSN, LCCE, FACCE

Tool box
- **Month Math ready-to-use sheet**
- **Written module or Internet/ intranet course**
- **Month Math Answer Key**

Preparation

1. Copy the Month Math ready-to-use sheet into the beginning of a written module or Internet/intranet course.
2. Copy the Month Math Answer Key into one of the last pages or screens of a written module or Internet/intranet course.
3. Reference the page number where the answer can be found on the Month Math ready-to-use sheet into the beginning of a written module or Internet/intranet course, so learners can check their answers.
4. Personalize the message at the end of the activity.
5. Continue with the information in the course or module.

Educator secrets
Thought-provoking activities such as these can warm up the thought process before the learners begin reading content information. You can also use this as a thought starter in a live class.

Implementation

1. Distribute written modules or ready your on-line course.
2. Answer any questions that may arise from the activity.

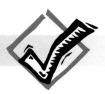

Month Math

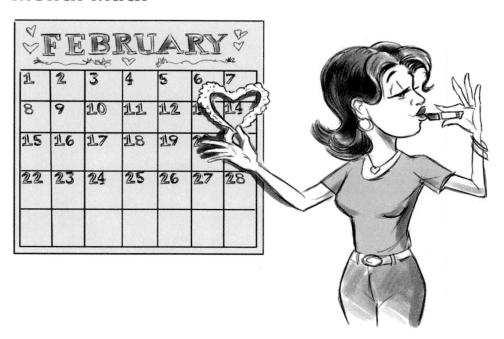

In a calendar year, 4 months have 30 days and 7 months have 31 days. How many months have 28 days?

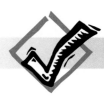

Month Math
ANSWER KEY

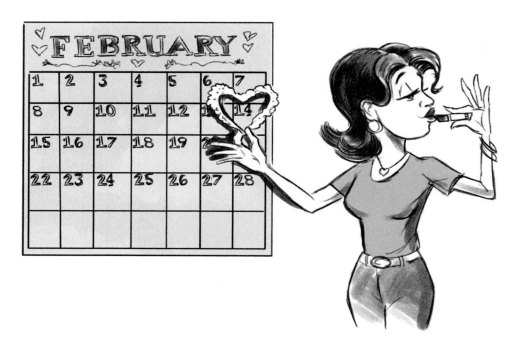

In a calendar year, 4 months have 30 days and 7 months have 31 days. How many months have 28 days?

ANSWER: All 12 months have 28 days. (Feel free to groan now.)

Sometimes we assume that the most obvious answer is the correct one. As this shows, we can use previously held knowledge to miss obvious facts. Of course every month has at least 28 days, but weren't we all thinking February? Do not jump to conclusions in this course. Good luck and keep thinking!

Alphabet Soup

Michele L. Deck, RN, MEd, BSN, LCCE, FACCE

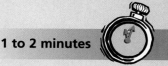

1 to 2 minutes

Preparation

1. Copy the Alphabet Soup ready-to-use sheet into the beginning of a written module or Internet/intranet course.
2. Copy the Alphabet Soup Answer Key into one of the last pages or screens of a written module or Internet/intranet course.
3. Reference the page number where the answer can be found on the Alphabet Soup ready-to-use sheet into the beginning of a written module or Internet/intranet course, so learners can check their answers.
4. Personalize the message at the end of the activity.
5. Continue with the information in the course or module.

Tool box
- **Alphabet Soup ready-to-use sheet**
- **Written module or Internet/ intranet course**
- **Alphabet Soup Answer Key**

Implementation

1. Distribute written modules or ready your on-line course.
2. Answer any questions that may arise from the activity.

Educator secrets
Thought-provoking activities such as these can warm up the thought process before the learners begin reading content information. You can also use this as a thought starter in a live class.

Alphabet Soup

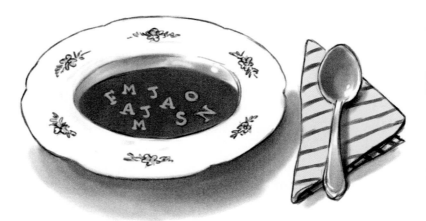

What is the next letter in the following sequence?

F M A M J J A S O N

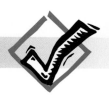

Alphabet Soup
ANSWER KEY

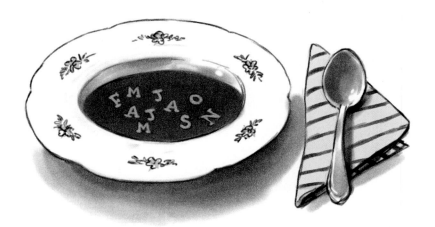

F M A M J J A S O N

The answer is **D**, for **December.** The letters stand for the first letter in the months of the year (except for January) in order.

February
March
April
May
June
July
August
September
October
November
December

I Know That

1 to 2 minutes

Michele L. Deck, RN, MEd, BSN, LCCE, FACCE

Tool box
- I Know That ready-to-use sheet
- Written module or Internet/ intranet course
- I Know That Answer Key

Preparation

1. Copy the I Know That ready-to-use sheet into the beginning of a written module or Internet/intranet course.
2. Copy the I Know That Answer Key into one of the last pages or screens of a written module or Internet/intranet course.
3. Reference the page number where the answer can be found on the I Know That ready-to-use sheet into the beginning of a written module or Internet/intranet course, so learners can check their answers.
4. Personalize the message at the end of the activity.
5. Continue with the information in the course or module.

Implementation

1. Distribute written modules or ready your on-line course.
2. Answer any questions that may arise from the activity.

Educator secrets
Thought-provoking activities such as these can warm up the thought process before the learners begin reading content information. You can also use this as a thought starter in a live class.

226

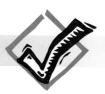

I Know That

DIRECTIONS: Please answer the following two questions:

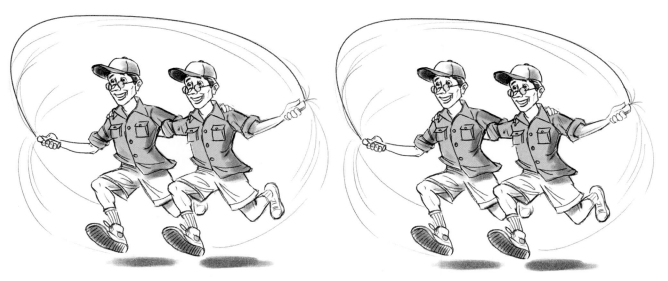

1. A pair of twins is how many people?

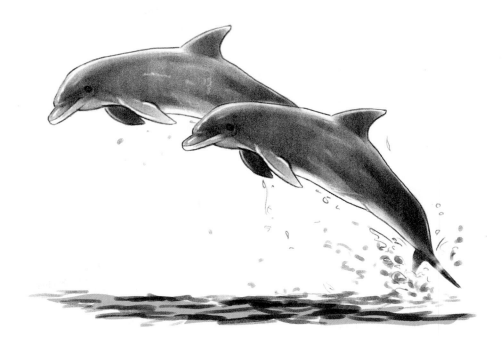

2. How many animals of each species did Moses take on the ark?

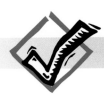

I Know That
ANSWER KEY

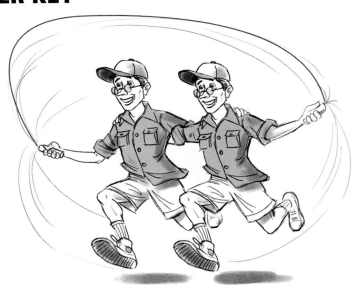

1. A pair of twins is how many people?
   The answer is two. A pair of twins is like a pair of shoes; one pair consists of two items or people. A twin is one person.

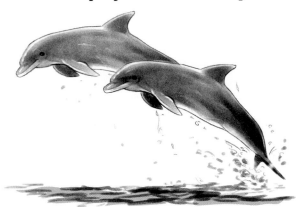

2. How many animals of each species did Moses take on the ark?
   The answer is none. Moses did not have an ark, Noah did. He's the person who took two of each species on the ark.

   Sometimes we don't fully pay attention to detail or even listen in our minds when we are reading. It might be that we notice something is wrong, yet we continue on as if ignoring it will fix it. Please read this information carefully, and if you notice something that stands out as incorrect to you, contact your instructor. Good luck!

Real-Life Geometry

Michele L. Deck, RN, MEd, BSN, LCCE, FACCE

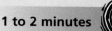

1 to 2 minutes

Preparation

1. Copy the Real-Life Geometry ready-to-use sheet into the beginning of a written module or Internet/intranet course.
2. Copy the Real-Life Geometry Answer Key into one of the last pages or screens of a written module or Internet/intranet course.
3. Reference the page number where the answer can be found on the Real-Life Geometry ready-to-use sheet into the beginning of a written module or Internet/intranet course, so learners can check their answers.
4. Personalize the message at the end of the activity.
5. Continue with the information in the course or module.

Tool box
- **Real Life Geometry ready-to-use sheet**
- **Written module or Internet/ intranet course**
- **Real Life Geometry Answer Key**

Implementation

1. Distribute written modules or ready your on-line course.
2. Answer any questions that may arise from the activity.

Educator secrets
Thought-provoking activities such as these can warm up the thought process before the learners begin reading content information. You can also use this as a thought starter in a live class.

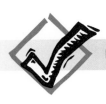

Real-Life Geometry

DIRECTIONS: Read the following scenario and come up with an explanation for it.

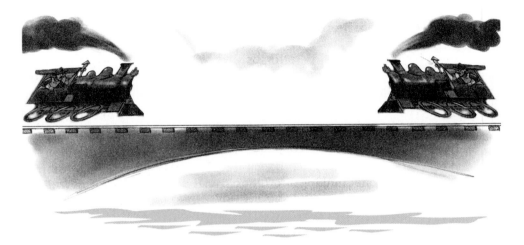

Two train tracks run parallel north and south, except for a short section where they meet and become one track. The meeting point is on a suspension bridge five miles long over a lake. One morning a train speeds onto the bridge heading north. Another train coming from the south also speeds onto the bridge. Neither train can stop on the bridge. Surprisingly, no collision takes place. How is this possible?

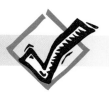

Real-Life Geometry
ANSWER KEY

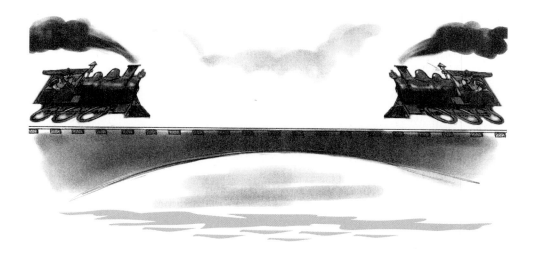

How is this possible?

It's possible because the trains were crossing the bridge at different times of the day, so there was no collision?

People sometimes jump to conclusions, based on limited data that they assume is all they need to understand a situation. Each of us have a different perceptual filter in our minds that color our perceptions. In this lesson, don't assume something is the case unless it is stated as such. Please begin the course now.

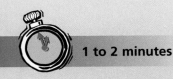

1 to 2 minutes

Weather or Not

Michele L. Deck, RN, MEd, BSN, LCCE, FACCE

Tool box

- **Weather or Not ready-to-use sheet**
- **Written module or Internet/ intranet course**
- **Weather or Not Answer Key**

Preparation

1. Copy the Weather or Not ready-to-use sheet into the beginning of a written module or Internet/intranet course.
2. Copy the Weather or Not Answer Key into one of the last pages or screens of a written module or Internet/intranet course.
3. Reference the page number where the answer can be found on the Weather or Not ready-to-use sheet into the beginning of a written module or Internet/intranet course, so learners can check their answers.
4. Personalize the message at the end of the activity.
5. Continue with the information in the course or module.

Implementation

1. Distribute written modules or ready your on-line course.
2. Answer any questions that may arise from the activity.

Educator secrets

Thought-provoking activities such as these can warm up the thought process before the learners begin reading content information. You can also use this as a thought starter in a live class.

232

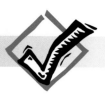

Weather or Not

DIRECTIONS: Please read the following scenario and answer the question posed at the end.

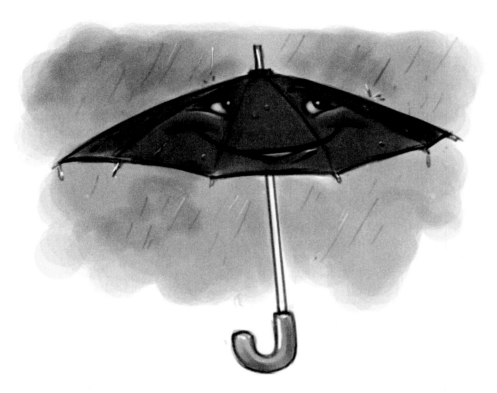

Stanley Shinyhead went for a walk without an umbrella. He did not wear a hat, nor did he stand under a tree. Yet, not one hair on his head got wet. How was this possible?

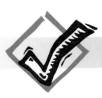

Weather or Not
ANSWER KEY

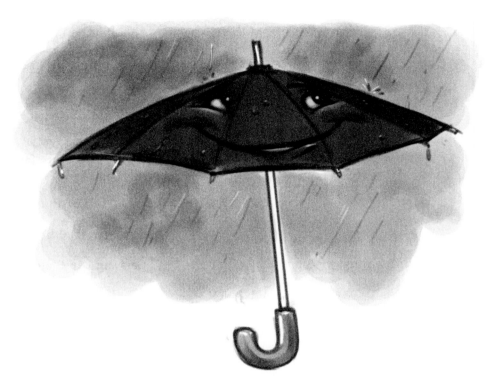

How was this possible?

It wasn't raining. Did you assume it was, or did you assume he was bald? Sometimes we fill in the blanks when it comes to situations when we don't have all the facts, but it seems right to guess at them. In this course, we encourage a basis in facts, not assumptions. Enjoy the course.

Baby Bulls Need Help

Michele L. Deck, RN, MEd, BSN, LCCE, FACCE

1 to 2 minutes

Preparation

1. Copy the Baby Bulls Need Help ready-to-use sheet into the beginning of a written module or Internet/intranet course.
2. Copy the Baby Bulls Need Help Answer Key into one of the last pages or screens of a written module or Internet/intranet course.
3. Reference the page number where the answer can be found on the Baby Bulls Need Help ready-to-use sheet into the beginning of a written module or Internet/intranet course, so learners can check their answers.
4. Personalize the message at the end of the activity.
5. Continue with the information in the course or module.

Tool box
- **Baby Bulls Need Help ready-to-use sheet**
- **Written module or Internet/ intranet course**
- **Baby Bulls Need Help Answer Key**

Implementation

1. Distribute written modules or ready your on-line course.
2. Answer any questions that may arise from the activity.

Educator secrets
Thought-provoking activities such as these can warm up the thought process before the learners begin reading content information. You can also use this as a thought starter in a live class.

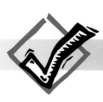

Baby Bulls Need Help

DIRECTIONS: Read the following scenario and answer the question.

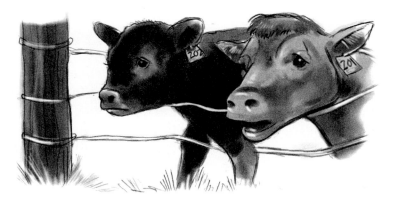

Two baby bulls are stuck in a fence. The mama Bull is waiting to the right of the following picture. The papa bull is off to the left of the picture. To which parent are the baby bulls most likely to go to get out of the fence?

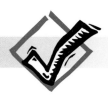

Baby Bulls Need Help
ANSWER KEY

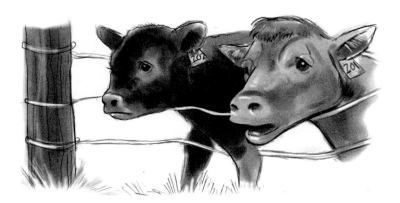

The baby bulls will go to the left to the papa bull. No such animal as a mama bull exists—only bulls (males) and cows (females). Therefore they would not be enticed to go to the right, even though the fence is in the way.

Pay attention to small details in this course. Many of you are familiar with this topic and may be tempted to skim through it. Please take the time to look at all the details because they do matter.

237

1 to 2 minutes

Math Mix-Up

Michele L. Deck, RN, MEd, BSN, LCCE, FACCE

Tool box

- **Math Mix-Up ready-to-use sheet**
- **Written module or internet/ Intranet course**
- **Math Mix-Up Answer Key**

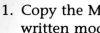

Educator secrets

Thought-provoking activities such as these can warm up the thought process before the learners begin reading content information. You can also use this as a thought starter in a live class.

Preparation

1. Copy the Math Mix-Up ready-to-use sheet into the beginning of a written module or Internet/intranet course.
2. Copy the Math Mix-Up Answer Key into one of the last pages or screens of a written module or Internet/intranet course.
3. Reference the page number where the answer can be found on the Math Mix-Up ready-to-use sheet into the beginning of a written module or Internet/intranet course, so learners can check their answers.
4. Personalize the message at the end of the activity.
5. Continue with the information in the course or module.

Implementation

1. Distribute written modules or ready your on-line course.
2. Answer any questions that may arise from the activity.

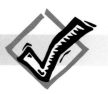

Math Mix-Up

DIRECTIONS: Pick a number between 1 and 9.

1. Multiply your number by 9.
2. If you have a two-digit number, add the single digits together. (Example: 24 would be 2 + 4 = 6)
3. Now, subtract 5 from your number.
4. With the number from above, change your number to a letter using this key:
   1 is an A
   2 is a B
   3 is a C
   4 is a D
   5 is an E
   6 is an F
   7 is a G
   8 is an H and so on

Think of a country that begins with the letter you received from the above key. Think of the last letter in the name of the country you picked. Select an animal whose name begins with the last letter of the country.

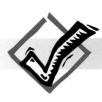

Math Mix-Up
ANSWER KEY

Actually, no kangaroos or koalas live in Denmark.

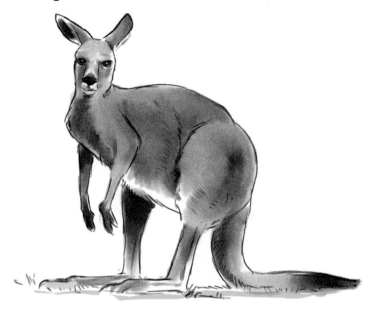

Are you surprised? If you did the math correctly, I should have been able to predict your answer. Because of extensive needs assessment, I have been able to predict what most people need to learn about this topic. I hope you find this course meaningful and relevant as predicted. Enjoy the information!

PART 6
Advice from Experience

Advice from Experience

Whether you are a new educator or a very seasoned one, you can always strive to make the learning experience productive for all of your learners. Early on in the process of becoming an educator, one discovers that knowing a topic well and being able to teach it well are two very different things. Both of these activities require different talents and skills that must be learned and improved upon.

A great learning experience involves both the educator and the participants using equal energy and being actively involved and interested. One cannot force others to learn—it is a choice and can be a fun experience that is full of discovery for everyone involved. It does not have to be dull, long, boring, and traditional. It can be what you, the educator, make it. It all depends on the approach you take, your teaching plan, your attitude, and the willingness of your learners. I like to create an atmosphere that makes the process of learning joyful, even if the content is serious and the learners' participation is *mandated.* This way the learners get so involved in the parts they like, that they must smile and talk to their peers in positive ways. They want to leave and use the new information and skills, because they see value in them. This joyful approach can be used in written modules, Internet/ intranet courses, and live classroom setups.

The ability to adapt your classes to a wide variety of people, places, and things is a challenge. I think the best skill an educator can have is the ability to "make lemonade" when life serves lemons. Try not to apologize when things go wrong. Instead, shift gears and move forward. If the learners have not seen your class before, they may never know a problem exists unless you tell them so, so don't. Pretend you are flexible and move on. Take another approach than the one planned. Have more than one way to teach everything so that if your hard drive dies, you still have the information in overheads or wall charts. If the videotape breaks, pull out your backup copy. When the computer system in computer class decides to go offline, announce to your group you have programmed these breaks in the day to offer them a chance to review. Invite them to form small teams and list everything they know so far about the computer that they have learned in class. Get to your room early to make sure no one has stolen all the chairs for a staff meeting down the hall. Give yourself permission to adapt as necessary and to be creative.

I'll never forget the first time I was given the opportunity to "make lemonade." I was traveling to Pittsburgh from my home in New Orleans to conduct a 2-day class on teaching others effectively. I carefully packed all my supplies, notes, and clothing, and I checked my luggage through to Pittsburgh. Because of mechanical problems with the connecting airplane, I didn't arrive until almost 2 AM. I went down to the baggage claim area of the airport to find nothing. My bags were lost, and I had nothing but the jeans, sweater, and tennis shoes that I had worn on the plane. I was such a travel rookie that I didn't even have a toothbrush with me! Luckily, the airline provided me with their overnight kit, which contained a toothbrush, toothpaste, and a comb. I went to my hotel in a panic, because even my notes were lost! I had only taught this 2-day class a few times previously and was still very note dependent. I remember I called my friend Doug, who was acting as my mentor and asked what I should do. He told me to get up early and see what I could find in the way of supplies at the hotel. He said to put the same dirty clothes on, go down to the meeting room, act like everything was perfect, and do the best I could. I told him as a female, a hairdo and makeup were a basic necessity, and I didn't have either! He convinced me to make lemonade on the spot. I found a deck of cards in the hotel gift shop, and a red-and-black marker supplied with the hotel flipchart. As I greeted suit-clad participants at the door, they looked at my outfit with curiosity (this was before business casual was invented) but came in anyway. I did the best job teaching that day I possibly could. I discovered a reward system and several activities to do with the playing cards that I thought up on the spot. At the end of the day, I called my friend to debrief. He suggested I go to a nearby store and buy a comparable outfit but no makeup or hairdo materials. I found a pair of white jeans and a blue sweater I still wear to this day. I continued to make the best of day 2, still without supplies. At the end of the course, I felt I had gotten to know each participant in a way I never had before, because I was totally focused on them and their needs without the distraction of high-tech audiovisuals, books of notes, and even my fashion look. I learned so much about myself that trip. I stretched and grew as an educator in those 2 days, and I never told one of the participants what had happened. Well, at least not then, but the story continues.

I was at the American Society for Training and Development (ASTD) Conference 3 years after my trip to Pittsburgh. I had on a chic business suit and was made up to look like a professional woman, standing in a booth in the exhibit hall. Three of the participants from my Pittsburgh class came up to me and were so excited to tell me how great the class was and how they had changed the way they taught because of our time together. However, one of three was speechless; she just kept staring at me. Finally, she said to me in front of the others, "Wow, Michele, you've had a beauty make-over haven't you? Look at your makeup and hairdo and the great suit! You go girl!" It was then I was able to explain to those three wonderful participants that my luggage was lost by the airlines and did not show up again for a week. I had to teach the class the best I could, making lemonade out of lemons. They looked stunned and admitted they thought my look was a bit odd but had no idea I was missing any notes, etc. They thought I taught extemporaneously without notes or high-tech visuals, and they were impressed with that. All of us left each other a little amazed. Since that time I have had multiple opportunities to live by this belief, and each time I have become a better person and educator for it. Therefore the next time you feel frustrated that things aren't perfect, think about making lemonade!

Every truly great educator I have met has been able to focus and connect with learners rather than over worry about themselves. These educators start with the end result in mind for their learners and figure out ways to get them from Point A to Point B. They look at the most interactive ways to teach so that results are achieved. They do not simply perform a content dump. Instead, they take their learners on a journey that has opportunities for reflection and practice. Sometimes educators must forge a new trail and try something new. In this case they must put their fears aside and move forward. In fact, one trait I have found consistently in successful educators and instructors is a sense of courage. They are not afraid to try something new to help their students learn. They may not even be experts at the topics they are asked to teach, but are willing to jump in and become knowledgeable about them. I remember a friend with clinical experience in psychiatric nursing who learned everything there was to know about central lines so that she could teach about them. She had never seen one in her clinical area, yet when charged with teaching it, she asked such great questions that we all learned. Her approach was fresh and unique, and even the assistive personnel who attended her classes left with a clear understanding of central lines. It took courage for her to step out of her comfort zone, learn something completely new, and then find a new approach to teach it.

This book is meant to be a tribute and collection of educators' courageous efforts to find unique approaches to teaching. Each one has been created and field-tested by a courageous educator and, for some, a group of courageous educators. They have shared their efforts so that everyone else doesn't have to reinvent the wheel. Give them a chance in your learning environment—whether it is live or virtual—and you will be surprised by the results. Your classes will stand out as different from others in the learners' experience, and they will remember you and your content years later. You will see improvement in students at all learning levels. The involving activities in this book will make it possible for even nonreaders to grasp the content. You and your participants will enjoy the learning experience more, and your evaluations will move from the center of the chart to the ends. Few people will remain neutral in class but will mentally be alert and present. I hope this book inspires you to create your own activities for learning so that a larger collection of creative ways to teach exists to further our profession. You can look forward to sharing the joy of discovery of new and effective ways to teach.

One last trait of very successful educators is that they never forget what it is like to stand in the learner's shoes. They seek opportunities to go to educational programs that develop their teaching skills. They remember what it feels like the night before their first clinical rotation in nursing school; they remember the joy of the first patient they were able to help and the sorrow of the first patient they grieved. They are connected to the important and life-touching experience that health care brings each and every day. They are creating the generations of nurses and health care providers who might very well take care of them in the future. It is a challenging job if done right, and it is not often a quick process. It requires commitment and dedication to teaching and reaching many diverse people in incredibly short periods of time. What you do makes a difference in people's lives every day. That is a joyful and humbling life's work, and we are privileged to do it. It is not for the faint hearted but instead for the blessed. I will never forget the first time I made a difference to a learner. Have you?

To assist educators in quickly locating an idea related to their content for ease of use, the following index of subjects is provided from all three teaching tools books:

- Vol. 1, *Instant Teaching Tools for Health Care Educators* (St. Louis, 1995, Mosby).
- Vol. 2, *MORE Instant Teaching Tools for Health Care Educators* (St. Louis, 1998, Mosby).
- Vol. 3, *Instant Teaching Tools for the New Millennium* (St. Louis, 2004, Mosby).

Note in which volume your activity appears, then the page number.

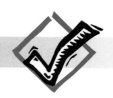

INDEX OF SUBJECTS

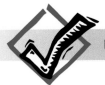

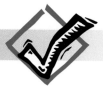

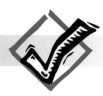

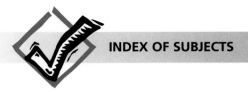

252